Workbook

Rau's Respiratory Care Pharmacology

Ninth Edition

Douglas S. Gardenhire, EdD, RRT-NPS
Director of Clinical Education
Division of Respiratory Therapy
School of Health Professions
Georgia State University
Atlanta, Georgia

Sandra T. Hinski, MS, RRT-NPS
Faculty, Respiratory Care Division
Gateway Community College
Phoenix, AZ

ELSEVIER

ELSEVIER

3251 Riverport Lane
St. Louis, Missouri 63043

Workbook for Rau's Respiratory Care Pharmacology ISBN: 978-0-323-29973-2
Copyright © 2016, Elsevier Inc. All rights reserved.
Previous editions copyrighted 2012, 2008, 2002.

All rights reserved. No part of this publication may be reproduced or transmitted in any form or by any means, electronic or mechanical, including photocopying, recording, or any information storage and retrieval system, without permission in writing from the publisher, except that, until further notice, instructors requiring their students to purchase Workbook for Rau's Respiratory Care Pharmacology by Douglas S. Gardenhire and Sandra T. Hinski, may reproduce the contents or parts thereof for instructional purposes, provided each copy contains a proper copyright notice as follows: Copyright © 2016, Elsevier Inc.

Details on how to seek permission, further information about the Publisher's permissions policies and our arrangements with organizations such as the Copyright Clearance Center and the Copyright Licensing Agency, can be found at our website: www.elsevier.com/permissions.

This book and the individual contributions contained in it are protected under copyright by the Publisher (other than as may be noted herein).

Notices

Knowledge and best practice in this field are constantly changing. As new research and experience broaden our understanding, changes in research methods, professional practices, or medical treatment may become necessary.

Practitioners and researchers must always rely on their own experience and knowledge in evaluating and using any information, methods, compounds, or experiments described herein. In using such information or methods they should be mindful of their own safety and the safety of others, including parties for whom they have a professional responsibility.

With respect to any drug or pharmaceutical products identified, readers are advised to check the most current information provided (i) on procedures featured or (ii) by the manufacturer of each product to be administered, to verify the recommended dose or formula, the method and duration of administration, and contraindications. It is the responsibility of practitioners, relying on their own experience and knowledge of their patients, to make diagnoses, to determine dosages and the best treatment for each individual patient, and to take all appropriate safety precautions.

To the fullest extent of the law, neither the Publisher nor the authors, contributors, or editors, assume any liability for any injury and/or damage to persons or property as a matter of products liability, negligence or otherwise, or from any use or operation of any methods, products, instructions, or ideas contained in the material herein.

Content Strategist: Sonya Seigafuse
Content Development Manager: Billie Sharp
Content Development Specialist: Charlene Ketchum
Publishing Services Manager: Hemamalini Rajendrababu
Project Manager: Umarani Natarajan

Printed in United States of America

Last digit is the print number: 9 8 7 6 5 4 3 2 1

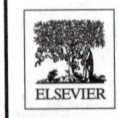 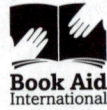

Working together to grow libraries in developing countries

www.elsevier.com • www.bookaid.org

Contents

Unit I: Basic Concepts and Principles in Pharmacology
1. Introduction to Respiratory Care Pharmacology, **1**
2. Principles of Drug Action **10**
3. Administration of Aerosolized Agents **22**
4. Calculating Drug Doses **35**
5. Central and Peripheral Nervous Systems **44**

Unit II: Drugs Used to Treat the Respiratory System
6. Adrenergic (Sympathomimetic) Bronchodilators **54**
7. Anticholinergic (Parasympatholytic) Bronchodilators **70**
8. Xanthines **79**
9. Mucus-Controlling Drug Therapy **89**
10. Surfactant Agents **99**
11. Corticosteroids in Respiratory Care **109**
12. Nonsteroidal Antiasthma Agents **120**
13. Aerosolized Antiinfective Agents **127**
14. Antimicrobial Agents **135**
15. Cold and Cough Agents **143**
16. Selected Agents of Pulmonary Value **150**
17. Neonatal and Pediatric Aerosolized Drug Therapy **158**

Unit III: Critical Care, Cardiovascular, and Polysomnography Agents
18. Skeletal Muscle Relaxants (Neuromuscular Blocking Agents) **166**
19. Diuretic Agents **176**
20. Drugs Affecting the Central Nervous System **184**
21. Vasopressors, Inotropes, and Antiarrythmic Agents **194**
22. Drugs Affecting Circulation: Antihypertensives, Antianginals, Antithrombotics **205**
23. Sleep and Sleep Pharmacology **216**

The Answer Key can be found by accessing http://evolve.elsevier.com/Gardenhire/Rau/respiratory

Reviewers

Lisa Conry, MA, RRT
Instructor, Respiratory Care
Spartanburg Community College
Spartanburg, SC

Margaret-Ann Carno, PhD, MBA, CPNP, ABSM, FNAP
Professor of Clinical Nursing and Pediatrics
Director RN to BS Completion Program
University of Rochester
School of Nursing
Rochester, NY

UNIT ONE BASIC CONCEPTS AND PRINCIPLES IN PHARMACOLOGY

1 Introduction to Respiratory Care Pharmacology

CHAPTER OUTLINE

Key Terms and Definitions
Naming Drugs
Sources of Drug Information
Sources of Drugs
Process of Drug Approval in the United States
Orphan Drugs
The Prescription
Respiratory Care Pharmacology: An Overview
Related Drug Groups in Respiratory Care
National Board for Respiratory Care (NBRC) Testing Questions
Case Study

CHAPTER OBJECTIVES

After answering the following questions, the reader should be able to:

1. Define *pharmacology*
2. Define *drugs*
3. Describe how drugs are named
4. List the different sources of drug information
5. List the various sources used to manufacture drugs
6. Describe the process for drug approval in the United States
7. Define *orphan drugs*
8. Differentiate between prescription drugs and over-the-counter drugs
9. Apply the various abbreviations and symbols used in prescribing drugs
10. Describe the therapeutic purpose of each of the major aerosolized drug groups
11. Identify related drug groups in respiratory care

KEY TERMS AND DEFINITIONS

Complete the following questions by writing the answer in the space provided.

1. Application of pharmacology to the treatment of pulmonary disorders and, more broadly, critical care is called a _____.

2. The study of drugs (chemicals), including their origin, properties, and interactions with living organisms, is called _____.

3. The time course and disposition of a drug in the body, based on its absorption, distribution, metabolism, and elimination, is called _____.

4. The mechanism of drug action by which a drug molecule causes its effect in the body is called _____.

5. The study of toxic substances and their pharmacologic actions, including antidotes and poison control, is called _____.

6. The name assigned to a chemical, when it appears that the chemical has therapeutic use and the manufacturer wishes to market the drug, is _____ _____.

7. A virus that causes the formation of syncytial masses in cells and may cause respiratory distress in young infants is called _____ _____ _____.

8. _____ _____ is an organism that causes *Pneumocystis* pneumonia in humans and is seen in immunosuppressed individuals, such as those infected with the human immunodeficiency virus (HIV).

9. The art of treating disease with drugs is called _____.

10. A _____ is the written order for a drug, along with any specific instructions for compounding, dispensing, and taking the drug.

NAMING DRUGS

Complete the following by writing the answer in the space provided.

11. A _____ name is given to an experimental chemical that shows potential as a drug.

12. The _____ name indicates the drug's chemical structure.

13. The _____ name is what the generic name becomes once it receives official approval.

14. The _____ name is the nonproprietary name (*example:* Motrin; Tylenol).

15. Fill in the following different names for the antiasthmatic drug zafirlukast.

    a. Chemical name _____

    b. Code name _____

    c. Official name _____

    d. Generic name _____

    e. Trade name _____

SOURCES OF DRUG INFORMATION

Complete the following questions by writing the answer in the space provided.

16. What is an official source of information about drug standards if you want to obtain information about medications, dietary supplements, and medical devices? The U.S. Food and Drug Administration (FDA) considers this book the official standard for drugs marketed in the United States.

    _____

17. This reference source has lots of color charts that identify drugs, lists manufacturers, and tells how the drugs work, when they are indicated and contraindicated, and possible side effects.

    _____

18. What subscription service provides monthly information on drug products and new releases?

    _____

SOURCES OF DRUGS

Complete the following question by writing the answer in the space provided.

19. Most of today's drugs come from chemical synthesis, but _____, _____, _____, and _____ also contain certain active ingredients for drugs.

PROCESS OF DRUG APPROVAL IN THE UNITED STATES

Complete the following questions by writing the correct term in the blank provided.

20. Provide a brief description of each of the phases involved in the investigational new drug (IND) approval process.

    a. Phase 1: _____

    b. Phase 2: _____

    c. Phase 3: _____

21. After a successful IND process, a New Drug Application (NDA) is filed with the FDA, and a detailed reporting system is in place for _____ months to track any problems that arise with the drug's use.

Match each of the following definitions with the correct classification of therapeutic potential by placing the letter of the best answer in the space provided.

22. _____ Important (significant) therapeutic gain over other drugs

23. _____ Modest therapeutic gain

24. _____ Important therapeutic gain, indicated for a patient with AIDS; fast-track

25. _____ Little or no therapeutic gain

A
AA
B
C

ORPHAN DRUGS

After each question, provide the correct answer.

26. Define the term *orphan drugs*.

27. When referring to orphan drugs, what does the term *rare* mean?

28. An orphan drug that respiratory clinicians use for the treatment of persistent pulmonary hypertension of newborns is called _____ _____.

29. Tobramycin, or TOBI, is an orphan drug used to treat _____ _____ in patients with cystic fibrosis (CF) or bronchiectasis.

30. An orphan drug used to prevent or treat respiratory distress syndrome in newborn infants is _____.

THE PRESCRIPTION

The prescription is the written order for a drug. It contains instructions for the pharmacist and patient about how to make, dispense, and take the drug.

Answer the following questions about the prescription.

31. Name the six parts of a prescription.

    a. _____

    b. _____

    c. _____

    d. _____

    e. _____

    f. _____

32. Give an example of an over-the-counter (OTC) drug.

33. True or False: The prescriber must write on the prescription that it is okay to use the generic form of the drug. _____

34. Use Table 1-3 in the textbook to match the following list of abbreviations with their meanings.

    a. qd   _____

    b. bid   _____

    c. et   _____

    d. cc   _____

    e. gtt   _____

    f. IM   _____

    g. L   _____

    h. mL   _____

    i. PO   _____

    j. q   _____

    k. prn   _____

    l. nebul _____

    A drop
    A spray
    And
    As needed
    By mouth
    Cubic centimeter
    Every
    Every day
    Every hour
    Every other day
    Four times daily
    Intramuscular
    Intravenous
    Liter
    Milliliter
    Nothing by mouth
    Three times daily
    Twice daily

m. NPO _____

n. qh _____

o. qod _____

p. qid _____

q. tid _____

r. IV _____

RESPIRATORY CARE PHARMACOLOGY: AN OVERVIEW

Using Table 1-4 in the textbook, provide the answers for questions 35 and 36.

Complete the following question by writing the correct terms in the blanks provided.

35. List five advantages of aerosolized agents given by inhalation.

    a. _____

    b. _____

    c. _____

    d. _____

    e. _____

36. Fill in the blank sections of the following table, which refers to common agents used in respiratory therapy.

Drug Group	Therapeutic Purpose	Agent
Adrenergic	a.	Albuterol
Anticholinergic	Relaxation of bronchoconstriction	b.
Mucoactive	c.	Mucomyst
Corticosteroid	Reduction of airway inflammation	d.
Antiasthmatic	e.	f.
Antiinfective	Elimination of infective agents	g.
Surfactant	h.	Infasurf
i.	Pulmonary hypertension	Treprostinil

RELATED DRUG GROUPS IN RESPIRATORY CARE

Complete the following questions by writing the answer in the space provided.

37. Drugs used to treat infections, such as antibiotics and antifungal drugs, are called _____ _____.

38. These agents paralyze people and are used in critical care. An example of this type of drug is Pavulon. _____ _____ _____.

39. A drug used to help reduce the effect of pain by affecting the central nervous system (*example:* morphine) is called a(n) _____.

40. Drugs that treat dangerous cardiac dysrhythmias (*example:* lidocaine) are called _____.

41. These drugs, used to treat high blood pressure and chest pain (*example:* β blockers, nitroglycerin), are called _____ _____ _____.

42. These agents help to keep blood from clotting (*example:* heparin). _____ _____ _____.

43. To rid the body of excess body fluid (whether in the lungs, heart, etc.), a(n) _____ would be administered.

44. Match the aerosolized drug group with the agent.

    1. _____ dornase alfa
    2. _____ zafirlukast
    3. _____ beractant
    4. _____ ribavirin
    5. _____ beclomethasone dipropionate
    6. _____ ipratropium bromide
    7. _____ epinephrine

    a. Antiinfective agent
    b. Antiasthmatic agent
    c. Mucoactive agent
    d. Anticholinergic agent
    e. Adrenergic agent
    f. Corticosteroid
    g. Exogenous surfactant

NATIONAL BOARD FOR RESPIRATORY CARE (NBRC) TESTING QUESTIONS

1. Animal studies are designed to accomplish which of the following?
   a. General effect on the organism
   b. Effects on specific organs
   c. Toxicology studies
   d. All the above

2. Studies involving human subjects occur during which stage of the drug approval process?
   a. Chemical identification
   b. IND approval
   c. NDA
   d. Internal review

3. Which of the following is the generic name for the antiasthmatic drug Accolate?
   a. Proventil
   b. Zafirlukast
   c. ICI 204,219
   d. ED-AA

4. If you are looking up a drug in a reference source that has color charts that identify drugs, lists manufacturers, and tells how the drugs work, you are looking in the
   a. *Hospital Formulary*
   b. *Hospital Reference Source*
   c. *Physicians' Desk Reference*
   d. *Drug Handbook*

5. Which of the following is an advantage of aerosolized agents by inhalation?
   a. Aerosol doses are larger than those used for the same purpose and given systemically.
   b. Aerosolized agents have more side effects than those given systemically.
   c. Aerosolized agents have a slower onset of action.
   d. Drug delivery is targeted to the respiratory system and is painless.

6. An order has been written for a patient to receive an aerosolized bronchodilator tid. This would indicate the patient should receive the treatment
   a. Four times a day
   b. Three times a day
   c. Once a day
   d. Every 3 hours

7. An agent that will relax bronchial smooth muscle and reduce airway resistance to improve ventilatory flow rate in chronic obstructive pulmonary disease (COPD) and asthma is
   a. Adrenergic
   b. Corticosteroid
   c. Antiinfective
   d. Mucoactive

8. A patient has been ordered to receive a corticosteroid. This could indicate the patient has a need for
   a. Bronchial smooth muscle relaxation
   b. Thinning of mucus
   c. Increase in lung compliance
   d. Reduction and control of inflammatory response in the airway

9. This is an agent that is used to rid the body of excess fluid that may accumulate in the lungs.
   a. Antiinfective
   b. Antithrombolytic
   c. Diuretic
   d. Anticoagulant

10. As you enter a patient's room, you notice a sign above the bed that reads "NPO." This would indicate
    a. Administer medications by mouth only
    b. Administer drugs by IV only
    c. Nothing by mouth
    d. No needlesticks

11. This legislation put more controls on biologic agents and toxins and was passed in 2002.
    a. Prescription Drug User Act
    b. Supplemental Drug and Enforcement Act
    c. Bioterrorism Act
    d. Amendment Act

12. A class of drugs including montelukast and zileuton is used to
    a. Reduce infection
    b. Prevent the onset of asthmatic response
    c. Help increase surface tension in the alveoli
    d. Reduce pulmonary hypertension

13. A specific aerosolized agent used to inhibit or eradicate specific infective agents in patients with CF is
    a. Pentamidine
    b. Tobramycin
    c. Ribavirin
    d. Zanamivir

14. A prostacyclin analog used to treat pulmonary hypertension would include
    a. Iloprost
    b. Zileuton
    c. Lucinactant
    d. Beractant

15. On reading a patient's medical history, it is learned the patient has a diagnosis of HIV infection. This would indicate the causative organism of the patient's pneumonia is likely
    a. *Pseudomonas aeruginosa*
    b. *Streptococcus aureus*
    c. *Haemophilus influenzae*
    d. *Pneumocystis carinii (jiroveci)*

CASE STUDY

An 8-year-old patient with CF has been admitted to the hospital. According to the patient's mother, this is his first hospital admission as a result of his CF. His CF has caused increased shortness of breath and more difficulty coughing up secretions. The following order has been written for respiratory care treatment:

Arterial blood gas stat
Albuterol 0.5 mL dil in 3.0 mL normal saline q4h and prn, et chest physical therapy p̄ nebul treatment qid
NPO 1h a chest physical therapy
Oxygen 2 L/min c̄ nasal cannula

1. Interpret this order, and identify the symbols and abbreviations used in this order.

2. During administration of the treatment, the mother of the patient asks why her son is receiving albuterol, because he has never used this medication. Explain.

   After 3 days of respiratory treatments, the patient has improved, and a new respiratory order has been written:

   Change albuterol and normal saline treatment.

3. What is wrong with this order?

2 Principles of Drug Action

CHAPTER OUTLINE

Key Terms and Definitions
Drug Administration Phase
Pharmacokinetic Phase
    Absorption
    Distribution
    Metabolism
    Elimination
    Pharmacokinetics of Inhaled Aerosol Drugs
Pharmacodynamic Phase
    Structure-Activity Relations
    Nature and Type of Drug Receptors
    Dose-Response Relations
Pharmacogenetics
National Board for Respiratory Care (NBRC) Testing Questions
Case Studies 1 and 2

CHAPTER OBJECTIVES

After answering the following questions, the reader should be able to:

1. Define key terms that pertain to principle of drug action
2. Define the *drug administration phase*
3. Describe the various routes of administration available
4. Define the *pharmacokinetic phase*
5. Discuss the key factors in the pharmacokinetic phase (absorption, distribution, metabolism, and elimination)
6. Describe the first-pass effect
7. Differentiate between systemic and inhaled drugs in relation to the pharmacokinetic phase
8. Explain the L/T ratio
9. Define the *pharmacodynamic phase*
10. Discuss the importance of structure-activity relations
11. Discuss the role of drug receptors
12. Discuss the importance of dose-response relations
13. Describe the importance of pharmacogenetics

KEY TERMS AND DEFINITIONS

Match the following definitions with their terms.

1. _____ A rapid decrease in response to a drug.

2. _____ A drug interaction that occurs from combined drug effects that are greater than if the drugs were given alone.

3. _____ Drug administration in any way other than by the intestine, most commonly by intravenous, intramuscular, or subcutaneous injection.

a. Parenteral
b. Transdermal
c. Inhalation
d. Enteral
e. Lung availability/systemic availability (L/T ratio)
f. Therapeutic index (TI)
g. Agonist

4. _____ Taking a substance, typically in the form of gases, fumes, vapors, mists, aerosols, or dusts, into the body by breathing in.

5. _____ Administration of a drug by use of the intestine.

6. _____ Difference between the minimal therapeutic and toxic concentrations of a drug; the smaller the difference, the greater the chance the drug will be toxic.

7. _____ A chemical or drug that binds to a receptor and creates an effect on the body.

8. _____ An abnormal or unexpected reaction to a drug, other than an allergic reaction, as compared with the predicted effect.

9. _____ The proportion of drug available from the lung, out of the total systemically available drug.

10. _____ Use of a patch on the skin to deliver a drug.

h. Synergism
i. Idiosyncratic effect
j. Tachyphylaxis

DRUG ADMINISTRATION PHASE

Complete the following questions by writing the correct term in the blank provided.

11. Tablets, capsules, and injectable solutions are examples of _____ _____ forms.

12. Oral, injection, and inhalation are examples of the _____ _____ _____.

13. List the five ways that a drug can be administered, and give one example of a common drug formulation.

Route of Administration of Drug

a. _____
b. _____
c. _____
d. _____
e. _____

Common Drug Formulation

a. _____
b. _____
c. _____
d. _____
e. _____

PHARMACOKINETIC PHASE

Complete the following questions by writing the correct term in the blank provided.

14. How the drug is absorbed, distributed, metabolized, and eliminated is the _____ phase.

15. How the drug causes an effect in the body is the _____ phase.

16. List the five layers of the lower respiratory tract that a drug must traverse before reaching the bloodstream for distribution into the body.

a. _____
b. _____
c. _____
d. _____
e. _____

Absorption

Fill in the blank with the type of absorption.

17. _____ occurs in the aqueous compartments of the body, such as interstitial spaces or within a cell.

18. _____ occurs across epithelial cells with lipid membranes. For a drug to be distributed in the body, it must cross the many epithelial membranes that have lipid membranes before it reaches the target organ.

19. _____ _____ occurs by special membrane-embedded carrier molecules transporting substances across membranes.

20. _____ is the incorporation of a substance into a cell by a process of membrane engulfment and transport of the substance to the cell interior in vesicles.

21. _____ is the proportion of the drug that reaches the systemic circulation.

22. Drugs that are _____ tend to be well absorbed into the bloodstream and across the blood-brain barrier.

Distribution

23. List the approximate volume in liters of each of the following major body compartments.

Compartment	Volume (L)
a. Vascular (blood)	_____
b. Interstitial fluid	_____
c. Intracellular fluid	_____
d. Fat (adipose tissue)	_____

24. What two factors can change the *volume of distribution* (V_D)?

    a. _____

    b. _____

Metabolism

Complete the following questions by writing the correct term in the blank provided.

25. The main organ for drug metabolism is the _____.

26. List the six common pathways for drug metabolism that are considered Phase 1.

    a. _____

    b. _____

    c. _____

    d. _____

    e. _____

    f. _____

27. The major enzyme system in the liver is the _____.

28. List the four most important isoenzyme families for drug metabolism.

    a. _____

    b. _____

    c. _____

    d. _____

29. Why is it important to know which particular cytochrome P450 (CYP) enzyme metabolizes a drug?

30. If a drug is highly metabolized by the liver, most of the drug's effect will be lost in passing into the liver before it even reaches the general circulation. This clinically important effect is called the _____-_____ effect.

31. List five routes of administration that can bypass the portal venous circulation and avoid the first-pass effect.

    a. _____

    b. _____

    c. _____

    d. _____

    e. _____

Elimination
Complete the following questions by writing the correct term in the blank provided.

32. The primary site for drug excretion is the _____.

33. _____ is a measure of the ability of the body to rid itself of a drug.

34. The time required for the plasma concentration of a drug to decrease by one-half is called the _____ _____.

35. True or False: Drugs with a short half-life must be given more frequently to maintain plasma levels.

36. In aerosol drug studies that involve bronchodilators, the _____ _____ is often represented, rather than the concentration of the drug.

Using Figure 2-5 in the textbook, provide the correct answer to the following questions.

37. Which drug would be considered fast acting but of short duration? _____

38. If a person needed a long-acting drug for nighttime duration, which one would meet the person's needs? _____

39. Which bronchodilator drug would be useful for maintenance therapy and has a duration of action of 4 to 6 hours? _____

Pharmacokinetics of Inhaled Aerosol Drugs

After each question, provide the correct answer(s) or fill in the blank(s).

40. What is the difference between a local drug effect and a systemic drug effect?

41. Give an example of a drug that causes a local effect and a drug that causes a systemic effect.

42. What percentage of an inhaled aerosol is swallowed?

43. What percentage of an inhaled aerosol reaches the lungs?

44. How much aerosol impacts in the mouth and contributes to the amount reaching the stomach?

45. True or False: If a swallowed aerosol drug is highly metabolized by the liver, then the systemic effects will be the result of lung absorption.

46. Lung availability/total systemic availability (L/T) basically tells how efficient _____ delivery is into the lung.

47. List four factors that increase the L/T ratio with inhaled drugs. What does each factor have in common?

    a. _____

    b. _____

    c. _____

    d. _____

PHARMACODYNAMIC PHASE

Complete the following question by writing the correct term in the blank provided.

48. What are *receptors*? _____.

Structure-Activity Relations

49. True or False: Because albuterol has receptors selective for the airway, it has little to no effect on heart rate _____.

50. The relationship between the chemical structure of a drug and its clinical effect or activity is termed the _____.

Nature and Type of Drug Receptors
Complete the following questions by writing the answer in the space provided.

51. List the mechanisms of drug receptor action that form the basis for the effects of two drug classes used in respiratory care.

52. List the four mechanisms for transmembrane signaling. Give an example of each.

   a. _____
   b. _____
   c. _____
   d. _____

53. What type of receptors mediate bronchodilation and bronchoconstriction in the airways in response to endogenous stimulation by the neurotransmitters epinephrine and acetylcholine?

54. A _____ is a term used to describe G proteins with a family of guanine nucleotide–binding proteins with a three-part structure.

Dose-Response Relations
Complete the following questions in the space provided.

55. The body's response to a drug is directly proportional to the drug's _____.

56. The _____ _____ of a drug is the greatest response that can be produced by the drug, so that even at a higher dose, no further response will occur.

57. Which drug is more potent? Drug A (median effective dose [ED_{50}] = 10 mg) or drug B (ED_{50} = 6 mg)?

58. The TI of Drug A is 3, and the TI of Drug B is 50. Which drug is safer?

59. A drug that binds to a receptor (affinity) and causes a response (efficacy) is called a(n) _____.

60. What is the difference between a full agonist and a partial agonist?

Define the following terms.
61. Chemical antagonism

62. Functional antagonism

63. Competitive antagonism

64. _____ _____ refers to when two drugs work against one another. For example, Drug A causes bronchodilation, and Drug B causes bronchoconstriction.

65. A special case of synergism, in which one drug has no effect but can increase the activity of the other drug, is an example of _____.

66. A drug that has the opposite effect, an unusual effect, or no effect compared with the effect it is supposed to have is said to be _____.

67. The term _____ describes an allergic or immune-related response to a drug that can be quite serious, even requiring ventilatory support.

68. The term _____ describes a decreasing intensity of response to a drug over time; over time, more of the drug is required to produce the same effect.

69. The term _____ describes a rapid decrease in responsiveness to a drug.

PHARMACOGENETICS

70. Define pharmacogenetics.

71. List three drugs that are used in respiratory and critical care that have been studied in pharmacogenetics.

    a. _____
    b. _____
    c. _____

NATIONAL BOARD FOR RESPIRATORY CARE (NBRC) TESTING QUESTIONS

1. Which of the following describes what a drug does to the body?
   a. Pharmacology
   b. Pharmacokinetics
   c. Pharmacodynamics
   d. Pharmacogenetics

2. Oral, injection, and inhalation are examples of:
   a. Drug dosage forms
   b. Routes of administration
   c. Pharmacokinetics
   d. Drug formulation

3. Which type of drug crosses the blood-brain barrier most easily?
   1. Nonionized
   2. Ionized
   3. Lipid soluble
   4. Water soluble
      a. 1 and 3
      b. 1 and 4
      c. 2 and 3
      d. 2 and 4

4. Which of the following is the main site of drug metabolism?
   a. Kidney
   b. Stomach
   c. Lung
   d. Liver

5. Which of the following is the main site of drug elimination?
   a. Intestine
   b. Stomach
   c. Kidney
   d. Liver

6. If a drug is administered more frequently than the half-life of the drug, which of the following may result?
   a. Synergy
   b. Accumulation
   c. Elimination
   d. Clearance

7. Which of the following drugs will cause a systemic effect in the body when administered?
   1. Oxymetazdine (Afrin)
   2. Zanamivir (Relenza)
   3. Inhaled morphine
   4. Inhaled insulin
      a. 1, 2
      b. 1, 4
      c. 2, 3, 4
      d. 1, 3, 4

8. Inhaled aerosols used in the treatment of pulmonary disease are intended to exert what effect on the lung?
   a. Local
   b. Systemic
   c. Kinetic
   d. Dynamic

9. The drug dose at which 50% of its maximal response occurs is termed the ED_{50}. This refers to what aspect of the drug?
   a. Maximal effect
   b. Half-life
   c. Therapeutic index
   d. Bioavailability

10. Which of the following terms is used to describe what happens when an individual experiences less response to a drug over time?
    a. Hypersensitivity
    b. Idiosyncratic
    c. Toxicity
    d. Tolerance

11. For any drug to cause any effect in the body, it must combine with which of the following?
    a. Target organ
    b. Another carrier drug
    c. Receptor
    d. Blood cell

12. When using a metered dose inhaler (MDI), approximately how much aerosol impacts in the mouth and contributes to the amount reaching the stomach?
    a. 70%
    b. 50%
    c. 10%
    d. 2%

13. What term describes the direct chemical interaction between drug and biologic mediator, which inactivates the drug?
    a. Functional antagonism
    b. Chemical antagonism
    c. Competitive antagonism
    d. Direct antagonism

14. Which of the following L/T ratios indicates more effective drug deposition into the lungs?
    a. 0.92
    b. 0.66
    c. 0.41
    d. 0.17

15. Devices for administration of inhaled drugs include which of the following?
    1. MDI
    2. Dry powder inhaler (DPI)
    3. Pneumatic nebulizer
    4. Ultrasonic nebulizer
       a. 1 and 2
       b. 2 and 3
       c. 2, 3, and 4
       d. 1, 2, 3, and 4

16. What could be done to increase the L/T ratio of an inhaled medication?
    a. Instruct the patient to breath fast and in a shallow manner.
    b. Use inhaled drugs with low first-pass metabolism.
    c. Use a reservoir device or holding chamber with an MDI.
    d. Instruct the patient to breathe slowly when using a DPI.

17. Which of the following is a drug that binds to a receptor and causes a response?
    a. Agonist
    b. Efficist
    c. Additive
    d. Antagonist

18. The effect of two drugs' being greater than the sum of the effect of each drug describes _____.
    a. Potentiation
    b. Additive
    c. Double whammy
    d. Synergism

19. The clinical effect of a bronchodilator is the result of which of the following?
    a. Systemic effects
    b. Drug deposition in the airway
    c. Oral absorption of the drug
    d. Systemic absorption through the stomach

20. The well-described variations among patients in their responses to drugs are increasingly traced to hereditary differences. When do these genetic or hereditary drug variations manifest themselves?
    a. When the patient is administered the drug
    b. During genetic testing
    c. During research of specific groups or individuals
    d. When the drug is discontinued

21. A patient being discharged from the hospital has an order for enteral administration of albuterol sulfate. This would indicate the drug is to be delivered by:
    a. Intravenous route
    b. Inhalation
    c. Mouth
    d. Suppository

22. The lower respiratory tract lining presents barriers to drug absorption. This barrier consists of which of the following:
    a. Type I pneumocyte
    b. Type II pneumocyte
    c. Capillary vascular network
    d. Epithelial lining

23. An order has been written for administration of a drug enterally. This indicates the drug can be given in which of the following forms:
    a. Tablet
    b. Patch
    c. Aerosol
    d. Paste

24. A patient needs a concentration of theophylline equaling 15 mg/L. It is determined that it will take a 525-mg dose to achieve this concentration. This dose is referred to as a:
    a. Loading dose
    b. Functional dose
    c. Primary dose
    d. Clinical dose

25. The following are sedative drugs with their plasma half-life indicated.

Drug	Plasma Half-Life (hr)
A	2.0
B	1.7
C	2.5
D	3.0

If you want a sedative that could be given less frequently, you would suggest which of the following?
a. Drug A
b. Drug B
c. Drug C
d. Drug D

CASE STUDY 1

R.E. is a 24-year-old man who has been brought to the emergency room by his wife because he has had a high fever with shaking chills for the past 24 hours. R.E. states that he has had bronchitis for the past couple of weeks. He is complaining of shortness of breath; his respiratory rate is 32 breaths/min; his heart rate is 108 beats/min. Auscultation reveals bilateral crackles in the lower lobes, with bilateral wheezing heard on inspiration. After examining him, both you and the physician agree that R.E. probably has pneumonia and will be admitted to the hospital for treatment. R.E. will need a bronchodilator for the wheezing and antibiotics for the pneumonia.

1. Which route(s) of administration would be best to deliver the bronchodilator and antibiotics? Explain your choices.

2. What drug would be best for his symptom of bilateral wheezing on inspiration?

R.E. has been admitted to the hospital, and it is now day 2 of his hospital stay. He has been receiving albuterol treatments by small volume nebulizer, and he is feeling much better. His respiratory rate is 18 breaths/min; his heart rate is 84 beats/min. The bilateral wheezing has been reduced, and now he has a slight wheeze bilaterally. R.E. comments that a lot of the medicine seems to be going out into the air and that he can taste it in the back of his throat. He asks you how much of the stuff really makes it into his lungs.

3. What do you tell him?

The doctor has ordered albuterol MDI to be used at home. You suggest that R.E. should also use a reservoir device with the MDI. The doctor does not understand why the reservoir device should also be used.

4. What would you tell the doctor?

CASE STUDY 2

Mrs. Gonzalez has entered the emergency department because of respiratory distress. After an hour of continuous albuterol treatment, a decision has been made to intubate the patient and place her on mechanical ventilation. The physician administers a short-acting neuromuscular paralyzing agent called *succinylcholine* and a mild sedative. The patient is now paralyzed. The respiratory therapist successfully orally intubates the patient and begins hand ventilation with a resuscitation bag attached to the endotracheal tube. After being placed on a mechanical ventilator, the patient is still paralyzed and not breathing on her own over the ventilator set rate. Both the physician and respiratory therapist believe this is a very unusual situation, because succinylcholine is fast acting and the patient should be paralyzed for only a few minutes, after which she should begin spontaneously breathing.

1. What has caused the prolonged paralysis of Mrs. Gonzales?

The patient has been on the ventilator for the past 20 minutes, and the patient is still paralyzed.

2. What should the respiratory therapist recommend?

3 Administration of Aerosolized Agents

CHAPTER OUTLINE

Key Terms and Definitions
Aerosol Therapy
Physical Principles of Inhaled Aerosol Drugs
Aerosol Devices for Drug Delivery
Age Guidelines for Use of Aerosol Devices
Endotracheal Tube Administration
National Board for Respiratory Care (NBRC) Testing Questions
Case Studies 1 and 2

CHAPTER OBJECTIVES

After answering the following questions, the reader should be able to:

1. Define terms that pertain to administration of aerosol agents
2. Define aerosol therapy
3. Select an appropriate aerosol medication nebulizer on the basis of particle size distributions
4. Discuss aerosol particle size and deposition in the lungs
5. Differentiate between the types of aerosol devices
6. Describe the clinical applications of aerosol devices
7. Recommend the use of various aerosol devices

KEY TERMS AND DEFINITIONS

Complete the following questions by writing the answer in the space provided.

1. The amount of solution that remains in the reservoir of a small volume nebulizer (SVN) once sputtering begins, causing a decrease in nebulization, is called the _____.

2. Testing in a laboratory is called _____ testing.

3. The diameter of a unit-density spherical particle having the same terminal settling velocity as the measured particle is the _____ _____ _____ _____.

4. An aerosol generator is also known as a(n) _____.

5. A nontoxic liquefied gas propellant used to administer medication from a metered dose inhaler (MDI) is a _____ _____.

6. An add-on device or extension for administration of a drug from an MDI is known as a _____. It describes both a spacer and a valved holding chamber.

7. The process of particles' depositing out of suspension to remain in the lung is called _____.

8. The depth within the lung reached by particles is referred to as _____.

9. The tendency of aerosol particles to remain in suspension is described as _____.

10. _____ _____ is testing done on animals or humans.

11. _____ refers to the size of particles in an aerosol, meaning many different particle sizes are present.

12. _____ refers to the size of particles in an aerosol, meaning the particles are the same sizes.

13. The particles in an aerosol are the same size. This is called _____.

14. Delivery of aerosol particles in the lung is called _____ _____.

15. _____ is suspension of liquid or solid particles in a carrier gas.

AEROSOL THERAPY

Complete the following questions by writing the answer in the space provided.

16. List three indications for the use of aerosol therapy.

    a. _____

    b. _____

    c. _____

17. List four advantages and disadvantages seen with aerosol delivery of drugs.

Advantages	Disadvantages
a. _____	a. _____
b. _____	b. _____
c. _____	c. _____
d. _____	d. _____

PHYSICAL PRINCIPLES OF INHALED AEROSOL DRUGS

18. The particle size of interest for pulmonary applications is in the range of _____ to _____ μm, and the *fine particle fraction* is considered to include particles smaller than _____ μm.

19. The particle size above and below which 50% of the mass of the particles is found (i.e., the size that evenly divides the mass of the particles in the distribution) is called the _____ _____ _____ _____ or MMAD.

20. The MMAD of aerosol particles that deposit in the nose and mouth is 10 to 15 μm. This size particle may be good for _____ sprays.

21. Aerosol particles with an MMAD range of _____ can make it to the lower respiratory tract. This is the appropriate size for the bronchoactive drugs that we use today.

22. Delivery of aerosols with a particle size of _____ is intended for the terminal airways and alveolar region.

23. Which SVN would you use for a patient for whom deposition is important in the upper airways and early airway generations?

24. Which aerosol particle size would be most helpful for a patient with perennial rhinitis?

25. What are three factors that influence aerosol deposition in the lung?

    a. _____

    b. _____

    c. _____

26. The settling of aerosol particles in the lung can increase with encouragement of a _____-_____.

27. Inhaled aerosol drugs not only are heterodisperse in size, but they also readily absorb moisture; in other words, they are _____.

AEROSOL DEVICES FOR DRUG DELIVERY

28. SVNs can be classified into three categories. These are:

    a. _____

    b. _____

    c. _____

29. Identify which nebulizer you would choose for the given clinical situation of a patient needing aerosol therapy.

    a. Older patient debilitated and in acute distress: _____

    b. A person who travels extensively: _____

    c. Drug dose may need to be modified based on patient's level of dyspnea: _____

    d. An infant who cannot hold his or her breath: _____

30. List three names also used to refer to a jet nebulizer.

    a. _____

    b. _____

    c. _____

31. Give a brief description of the following types of nebulizers.
    a. Jet nebulizer with a 6-inch reservoir tube

    b. Nebulizer with a collection bag

c. Breath enhanced nebulizer

d. Breath actuated nebulizer

32. Circle the correct answer: Because of significant evaporation of aqueous solution in a gas powered nebulizer, drug solute can become (increasingly/decreasingly) concentrated.

33. How does a mesh nebulizer work?

34. For efficient operation and relatively brief treatments (≤5 minutes), a filling volume of _____ is recommended.

35. With a filling volume of 5 mL, the flow rate should be between _____ and _____.

36. An SVN can be powered using either _____ or _____.

37. Explain why should a mouthpiece be used instead of a face mask for aerosol drug administration.

38. Regardless of the type of device interface used during aerosol therapy, how should you instruct your patients to breathe during aerosol therapy?

39. Higher-viscosity antibiotic solutions of gentamicin or carbenicillin require _____-_____ L/min power gas flow rates to produce suitably small aerosol particles for inhalation with some jet nebulizers.

40. Match the following drug to the approved nebulizer.
    1. _____ Bronchodilator
    2. _____ Pentamidine
    3. _____ Tobramycin
    4. _____ Pulmozyme
    5. _____ Ribavirin

    a. Pari LC
    b. No specific nebulizer
    c. Pari Baby
    d. Small-particle aerosol generator (SPAG)
    e. Marquest Respirgard II

41. Dr. Santiago always orders an SVN for his patient receiving aerosol administration. What are three advantages you could explain to him regarding why the patient could benefit from drug delivery with pressurized MDI (pMDI)?

   a. _____

   b. _____

   c. _____

42. Label the six components of an MDI.

43. Chlorofluorocarbon (CFC) propellant has been replaced by _____ propellant.

44. Name the types of pMDIs.

   a. _____

   b. _____

   c. _____

45. The hydrofluoroalkane (HFA) versions of pMDI have a more "_____" spray temperature compared with CFC spray.

46. Why should a reservoir device be used when delivering inhaled corticosteroids?

47. The most common error noted is the failure to coordinate inhalation, and actuation of the inhaler is _____ - _____ incoordination.

48. Describe the instructions you would give a patient for the correct use of their Combivent Respimat soft-mist inhaler.

49. If the pMDI has not been used for several days, what should be done to prime the valve?

50. After aerosol administration of a corticosteroid, what should you instruct your patient to do?

51. If you use both a bronchodilator and a corticosteroid, inhale the bronchodilator first and wait _____ to _____ minutes before inhaling the corticosteroid.

52. What is the most common error when using a pMDI?

   _____

53. What would you tell a patient about how to identify the need to clean the pMDI?

54. What are two ways canister fullness can be monitored?

   a. _____

   b. _____

55. Describe each of the following accessory devices for use with pMDI.
    a. Reservoir device
    b. Spacer
    c. Valved holding chamber

56. When using a spacer or holding chamber with collapsing bag, you should open the bag to its fullest size. The pMDI should actuate _____ inspiration.

57. What is a DPI?

58. The flow rate needed to disperse the drug of a DPI is _____.

59. List three categories of DPI inhalers.

   a. _____

   b. _____

   c. _____

60. List three factors that affect DPI performance and drug delivery.

   a. _____

   b. _____

   c. _____

61. With any DPI, it is absolutely essential that patients not _____ into the device before inhaling; in all devices, including the Diskus, the drug powder is exposed once the device is activated.

62. If a patient is using a pMDI and a DPI, what difference in the force of inhalation would need to be emphasized between the two devices?
    a. pMDI

    _____

    b. DPI

    _____

63. If powder remains in the chamber of a unit dose DPI inhaler, what should the patient do?

AGE GUIDELINES FOR USE OF AEROSOL DEVICES

64. Match the following aerosol systems to the appropriate age.

   1. _____ SVN
   2. _____ MDI
   3. _____ MDI with reservoir
   4. _____ MDI with reservoir and mask

   a. More than 5 years of age
   b. Neonate or older
   c. More than 4 years old
   d. Up to 2 years old
   e. Up to 4 years old

5. _____ MDI with endotracheal tube (ETT)

6. _____ Breath actuated MDI

7. _____ DPI

ENDOTRACHEAL TUBE ADMINISTRATION

65. Pediatric patients receiving aerosolized medications while undergoing mechanical ventilation may have a lower percentage of drug delivered because their _____ _____ is narrower.

66. Where should the SVN be placed in a patient receiving mechanical ventilation to improve aerosol delivery?

67. The _____-_____ _____ should be bypassed when delivering aerosolized medication to a patient receiving mechanical ventilation.

68. The use of a less dense gas, such as a _____-_____ mixture, can increase particle deposition.

69. When using an MDI, timing the actuation of the aerosol device with precise inspiration by the ventilator may increase drug delivery by _____.

70. List three variables present when administering aerosol drug by SVN or MDI to intubated, mechanically ventilated patients.

   SVN

   a. _____

   b. _____

   c. _____

   MDI

   a. _____

   b. _____

   c. _____

NATIONAL BOARD FOR RESPIRATORY CARE (NBRC) TESTING QUESTIONS

1. Aerosol therapy is used for which of the following purposes?
   1. Humidification of inspired gases
   2. Improving mobilization and clearance of secretions
   3. Augmenting alveolar ventilation
   4. Delivery of medication
      a. 2 and 3 only
      b. 1 and 4 only
      c. 1, 2, and 4 only
      d. 1, 2, 3, and 4

2. Which of the following are advantages of delivering medication using the aerosol versus systemic route of administration?
   1. Smaller doses are required.
   2. Onset of action is quicker.
   3. Side effects are fewer.
   4. Drug delivery is targeted to the respiratory system.
      a. 1 and 3 only
      b. 2, 3, and 4 only
      c. 1, 3, and 4 only
      d. 1, 2, 3, and 4

3. Which particle size is optimal for aerosol deposition in the terminal airways?
   a. More than 10 μm
   b. 5 to 10 μm
   c. 2 to 5 μm
   d. 0.8 to 3 μm

4. Nasal spray for use for perennial rhinitis has a particle size of which of the following?
   a. More than 10 μm
   b. 5 to 10 μm
   c. 2 to 5 μm
   d. Less than 0.8

5. Which aerosol delivery device operates on the piezoelectric principle?
   a. SVN
   b. SPAG
   c. DPI
   d. ultrasonic nebulizer (USN)

6. A type of nebulizer that uses a plate with multiple apertures and moves the medication through a fine mesh is called:
   a. SVN
   b. SPAG
   c. DPI
   d. Vibrating mesh

7. Which of the following aerosol delivery devices requires the patient to be able to generate an inspiratory flow rate of 30 to 90 L/min?
   a. USN
   b. SPAG
   c. MDI
   d. DPI

8. Which of the following is used to deliver the medication delivery in the Respimat inhaler?
   a. CFC
   b. HFA
   c. A tension spring
   d. Compressed gas

9. The greatest loss of drug with use of a SVN is primarily the result of:
   a. Exhaled medication into the atmosphere
   b. Impaction in the mouth
   c. Reduced deep breathing
   d. Drug remaining in the nebulizer

10. How much of the total drug dose is delivered to the lower respiratory tract of the lung, regardless of the delivery device used?
    a. 10% to 15%
    b. 30% to 40%
    c. 50% to 55%
    d. More than 55%

11. The MMAD of aerosol particles that deposit within the nose and mouth is:
    a. More than 10 μm
    b. 2 to 3 μm
    c. 1 to 2 μm
    d. More than 1 μm

12. For an aerosol to affect the lower respiratory tract of a patient with expiratory wheezing, you would want to use an SVN that delivered aerosol particle sizes in the range of:
    a. 10 to 15 μm
    b. 20 to 25 μm
    c. 1 to 5 μm
    d. 0.5 to 1.0 μm

13. What happens to the amount of drug in a nebulizer when diluent is added?
    a. The amount of drug stays the same.
    b. The concentration is tripled.
    c. The volume is reduced.
    d. The concentration is doubled.

14. With a filling volume of 5 mL in an SVN, the flow rate of the nebulizer should be set to:
    a. 4 L/min
    b. 4 to 5 L/min
    c. 6 to 8 L/min
    d. More than 10 L/min

15. When sputtering of the nebulized medication in an SVN occurs, shaking or agitating the SVN will do which of the following to the drug solution delivery?
    a. Increase the volume of drug solution
    b. Decrease the volume of drug solution
    c. Increase the drug solution concentration and delivery of the drug
    d. Have no effect on delivery of the drug solution

16. Which of the following is not a component of an MDI?
    a. Flow rate control
    b. Metering valve
    c. Propellant
    d. Drug

17. To prevent loss of dose when storing an HFA-propelled MDI canister of a drug, you should:
    a. Shake the MDI before storing it
    b. Store the canister in a valve-up position
    c. Give two puffs before storing the canister
    d. Store the canister on its side

18. When instructing a patient in the use of an MDI that delivers corticosteroids, to reduce oropharyngeal impaction of corticosteroids, you would tell the patient:
    a. To use an open mouth technique when inhaling the medication
    b. To use a closed mouth technique when inhaling the medication
    c. To inhale first and then give the puff of medication
    d. To use a spacer device or holding chamber

19. The term used to describe the loss of propellant from the metering valve of an MDI is:
    a. Creaming
    b. Loss of prime
    c. Actuation
    d. Crystallization

20. When instructing a patient in the use of a holding chamber, when should the patient actuate the pMDI?
    a. At the end of inspiration
    b. In the middle of inspiration
    c. Right before inspiration
    d. All of the above are correct related to actuation timing

21. Which of the following statements is true concerning delivery of a medication during mechanical ventilation of a child or adult?
    a. Using an MDI with a spacer device is better than using an SVN.
    b. Using an MDI without a spacer device is better than using an SVN.
    c. An SVN is better than an MDI with a spacer device.
    d. There is no difference between the use of an SVN and MDI with a spacer device.

22. To improve aerosol delivery during mechanical ventilation, an SVN should be placed:
    a. Directly on the endotracheal tube
    b. Between the Y adapter and the endotracheal tube
    c. After the humidifier, but as close to the ventilator and away from the circuit Y as possible
    d. Directly behind the heat-moisture exchanger on the inspiratory side of the patient circuit

23. A patient wants to know which of the following is the best way to determine when a pMDI is approaching its last dose:
    a. Placing the MDI in a hot water bath to see whether it floats
    b. Using a pMDI with an integrated dose counter
    c. Shaking the pMDI
    d. Weighing the pMDI

24. Which of the following aerosol delivery devices could be used for a child 6 months of age and admitted to the emergency department (ED) with a diagnosis of bronchiolitis?
    a. MDI
    b. DPI
    c. SVN
    d. Breath actuated MDI

25. When administering aerosol agents to a mechanically ventilated patient with a heat-moisture exchanger in place, the respiratory therapist should:
    a. Increase the inspiratory flow rate of the ventilator during the treatment
    b. Bypass the heat-moisture exchanger
    c. Place the aerosol device within 10 cm of the ETT
    d. Only administer the aerosol agent with an SVN

26. The most common error when using a pMDI is:
    a. Failure to coordinate actuation of MDI with inhalation
    b. Too rapid an inspiratory flow
    c. Inadequate shaking of MDI before use
    d. Actuation of MDI at total lung capacity

27. A patient on mechanical ventilation has been ordered to receive four puffs of a corticosteroid inline through the ventilator. How much time should be given between puffs to allow the valve to refill?
    a. 2 seconds
    b. 20 to 30 seconds
    c. 8 seconds
    d. No waiting is needed between puffs

28. A patient has been ordered to receive a bronchodilator and corticosteroid MDI. Which of the following is the correct method of administration of these drugs?
    a. Use the corticosteroid first, followed immediately by the bronchodilator.
    b. Use the corticosteroid first, then wait 20 to 30 seconds, and then use the bronchodilator.
    c. Use the bronchodilator first, followed immediately by the corticosteroid.
    d. Use the bronchodilator first, wait 1 to 2 minutes, and then use the corticosteroid.

29. Which of the following are critical steps in use of the closed mouth technique with pMDI?
    1. Warm the pMDI canister to hand temperature.
    2. Shake the inhaler.
    3. Prime the pMDI into the air.
    4. Have the patient exhale all the way out before administration of pMDI.
        a. 1, 2, and 3 only
        b. 2, 3, and 4 only
        c. 1, 3, and 4 only
        d. 1, 2, 3, and 4

30. While administering MDI treatment with a valved holding chamber, you hear a "whistling" sound. You would tell the patient to:
    a. Not to exhale into the holding chamber
    b. Take a deeper breath before actuation
    c. Take a slower inspiratory breath
    d. After a deep breath, hold the breath longer

CASE STUDY 1

Professor Craig, a 38-year-old man with a history of asthma, presents to the ED with a chief complaint of shortness of breath and coughing. His respiratory rate is 34 breaths/min, he is wheezing on both inspiration and expiration throughout both lung fields, and he has accessory muscle usage. He is unable to perform a peak expiratory flow rate maneuver. He complains of anxiety and is diaphoretic, his heart rate is 148 beats/min, and his oxygen saturation is 92% on room air. He is coughing up thick, white, foamy secretions. Oxygen is ordered for Professor Craig by nasal cannula at 2 L/min, as well as aerosol therapy with albuterol.

1. On the basis of this patient's presentation, what would be your recommendation for the choice of aerosol delivery device?

2. What is your rationale for making this selection?

3. The patient has a total medication volume in the nebulizer of 5 mL. What would be the appropriate flow rate to run the nebulizer? What compressed gas would you choose to power the device? Why?

4. When administering the medication nebulizer, what else could be emphasized to the patient that would help increase lung dose?

It is now 48 hours later. The wheezing has subsided considerably and is now heard slightly on expiration. Professor Craig has a respiratory rate of 22 breaths/min, oxygen saturation is 97% on room air, and his heart rate is 96 beats/min. He states that he is not experiencing shortness of breath and in general is feeling better. The patient has been ordered to receive a pMDI corticosteroid and a pMDI bronchodilator.

5. How would you instruct the patient in the administration of these drugs regarding which one should be given first?

6. Does he need a reservoir device? Why or why not?

7. Professor Craig has never used a pMDI and would like to know how he would know when the pMDI is close to the last puff?

CASE STUDY 2

Timmy is a 13-year-old patient and has been diagnosed with cystic fibrosis (CF). As part of his respiratory therapy, he has been ordered to receive various respiratory medications.

1. You have decided to administer these medications with a manual breath actuated jet nebulizer. Because the patient has never used this nebulizer before, how would you instruct Timmy on how to use this device?

2. Because Timmy will be using this nebulizer at home, what would you tell him concerning how often to clean the nebulizer and what should be used to clean the nebulizer?

3. The respiratory therapist believes it is also important that, at least once per week, the nebulizer should be disinfected. What would you tell Timmy is a way to disinfect the nebulizer?

4. After disinfecting the nebulizer, what should the respiratory therapist tell Timmy about the type of solution to use for rinsing the parts of the nebulizer?

5. Timmy tells you that another family whose child also has CF told him that white vinegar and hot water can also be used to disinfect his equipment, and it is a cheap way of doing it because vinegar is relatively inexpensive. What should the respiratory therapist tell Timmy about this method of disinfection?

4 Calculating Drug Doses

CHAPTER OUTLINE

Key Terms and Definitions
Calculating Doses from Prepared-Strength Liquids, Tablets, and Capsules
    Calculating with Proportions
    Drug Amounts in Units
    Calculations with a Dosage Schedule
    Additional Examples of Calculations with Prepared-Strength Drugs
Calculating Doses from Percentage-Strength Solutions
    Solutions by Ratio
    Solving Percentage-Strength Solution Problems
National Board for Respiratory Care (NBRC) Testing Questions
Case Studies 1, 2, and 3

CHAPTER OBJECTIVES

After answering the following questions, the reader should be able to:

1. Define key terms pertaining to calculating drug dose
2. Use the metric system
3. Calculate drug doses, using proportions
4. Calculate drug doses, using percentage-strength solutions

KEY TERMS AND DEFINITIONS

Complete the following questions by writing the answer in the space provided.

1. The amount of solute in a solution, usually expressed as a percentage, is called the _____.

2. The amount of solute that is in a solution containing 100 parts is the _____.

3. A physically homogeneous mixture of two or more substances is called a(n) _____.

4. A _____ is a substance that is dissolved in a solution.

5. A substance, usually a liquid, that is used to make a solution is called a _____.

6. The amount of drug that is needed, based on a patient's weight, is called _____.

To do drug calculations, you've got to use the metric system. (*Hint:* See Table 4-1 in the textbook.) Warm up with a few practice conversions:

7. 51 cm = _____ mm

8. 33 g = _____ mg

9. 24 mL = _____ L

10. 17 m = _____ cm

11. 68 kg = _____ g

12. 2 teaspoons = _____ drops

13. How many drops are in 1.0 mL? _____

One cubic centimeter (cc) equals 1 mL, so it is best to convert drops to milliliters and draw up medications in a small syringe, such as a tuberculin syringe. All drops are not created equal! The size of the opening and the properties of the liquid can influence the size of the drop.

14. A physician orders 1 teaspoon of a medication. How many milliliters does this equate to?

15. If a patient drank 4 cups of water, it would equal _____ fluid ounces.

16. A baby weighing 2500 g would weigh _____ kg.

17. If you had to give 0.001 L of a drug, you could draw it up in a tuberculin syringe, because you would only be giving _____ mL of the drug.

18. Levels of drug in the blood typically have units of measurement of _____ /mL.

CALCULATING DOSES FROM PREPARED-STRENGTH LIQUIDS, TABLETS, AND CAPSULES

Calculating with Proportions

19. Drug A comes in 200-mg tablets. A dose of 500 mg/day is prescribed. How many tablets should the patient take?

20. You are ordered to give 6 mg of dextromethorphan hydrobromide. How many milliliters of dextromethorphan hydrobromide should be given?

21. If there is 100 mg of drug in 50 mL of elixir and you want to give a 10-mg dose, how many milliliters of elixir should be given?

Drug Amounts in Units

22. How many milliliters do you need to give to deliver 650 U of heparin?

23. Insulin has a standard preparation of 1 unit = _____ mg.

Calculations with a Dosage Schedule

24. A mother of a child receiving albuterol syrup has a prepared mixture of 2 mg/5 mL, and the schedule requires 1 mg/kg. How much syrup is needed for a 25-kg child?

25. Quick! How many grams is 25 kg? _____

Additional Examples of Calculations with Prepared-Strength Drugs

26. If you have 10 mg/1 mL of morphine in an ampoule for injection, how much is needed to give a 2.0-mg dose intravenously?

27. A dosage schedule of a surfactant calls for 4 mL/kg of body weight for a 1200-g newborn infant. How many milliliters of surfactant will you need to administer?

28. A premature newborn weighs 1000 g. What dose of drug is needed that has a prepared strength of 100 mg/5 mL and a dosing schedule of 100 mg/kg?

CALCULATING DOSES FROM PERCENTAGE-STRENGTH SOLUTIONS

Respiratory therapists often calculate drug doses using solutions and percent strength.

29. To achieve a homogeneous solution, a _____ is dissolved in a _____.

Solutions by Ratio

30. What percent strength is a 1:100 solution of a drug?

Solving Percentage-Strength Solution Problems

31. How many milligrams of active ingredient are in 5 mL of a 1:250 drug?

32. A patient needs 3 mL of 10% Mucomyst, but only 20% Mucomyst is available. How much 20% Mucomyst should be used?

33. If you have 2.5 mL of a 20% solution and mix it with 2.5 mL of normal saline for a total of 5 mL, what will be the percent solution?

34. Although the definition of percentage strength in solution involves grams or milliliters, the amount of active ingredient in most nebulized drug solutions is in _____.

35. Complete the following medication calculations

Percent Strength (%)	Drug Amount (mg/mL)
a. 20%	_____
b. _____	100
c. 0.5	_____
d. 0.05	_____

36. Convert from gram to percent strength to mg/mL

Grams	Percent Strength	Drug Amount (mg/mL)
a. 0.001	0.1	_____
b. 0.002	_____	2
c. _____	0.3	3

37. If you have 2 mL of a 1% solution of a drug, how many milligrams is the active ingredient?

39. What is the amount of active ingredient in 0.5% strength albuterol that has a usual dose of 0.5 mL?

(Using equation for percentage strength on page 70 of the textbook)
40. Albuterol has 0.5% strength; what is the drug amount in mg/mL?

41. If you have a drug that is available as 2 mg/mL, what is the percent strength?

NATIONAL BOARD FOR RESPIRATORY CARE (NBRC) TESTING QUESTIONS

1. The respiratory care practitioner (RCP) is asked to add 1 g of metaproterenol to 100 mL of aqueous solvent. This will result in which of the following concentrations?
   1. 1:1000
   2. 0.01
   3. 1:100
   4. 1%
      a. 1 and 2 only
      b. 2 and 3 only
      c. 3 and 4 only
      d. 1 and 4 only

2. You are asked to administer 1 mL of a 1% solution of a drug to an asthmatic patient. How many milligrams of drug is this?
   a. 1 mg
   b. 10 mg
   c. 100 mg
   d. 1000 mg

3. The physician's order reads, "Administer 5 mg of metaproterenol via small volume nebulizer (SVN)." How many milliliters of a 1:100 solution should be used?
   a. 0.5
   b. 1
   c. 1.5
   d. 2

4. The RCP is asked to dilute 100 mL of a 2% solution of beclomethasone to a 1% solution. How many milliliters of water must be added to the original mixture to produce the desired concentration?
   a. 100
   b. 50
   c. 200
   d. 150

5. How many milliliters of water are needed to dilute 10 mL of a 20% solution of acetylcysteine to a 5% concentration?
   a. 40
   b. 60
   c. 50
   d. 20

6. The physician's order reads, "Instill 5 mL 5% NaHCO$_3$ q4h and prn." The pharmacy has 50-mL ampoules of an 8.4% solution. How many milliliters of distilled water must be added to make a 5% solution?
   a. 10
   b. 21
   c. 34
   d. 42

7. The physician's order reads, "Administer 75 mg Decadron via hand-held nebulizer." How many milliliters of a 2.5% solution should you use?
   a. 2.2
   b. 0.5
   c. 3
   d. 1.5

8. The amount of drug that is needed, based on a patient's weight, is called:
   a. Solution
   b. Body weight proportion
   c. Schedule
   d. Active ingredient

9. What is the percent strength of a drug available at 50 mg/mL?
   a. 1
   b. 5
   c. 10
   d. 15

10. The usual dose of albuterol sulfate is 0.5 mL of a 0.5% strength solution. How many milligrams is this?
    a. 5.0
    b. 2.5
    c. 1.25
    d. 0.50

11. Surfactant has been ordered to be delivered to a premature newborn infant weighing 1.2 kg. What dose should be delivered for a dosage schedule of 5 mL/kg of body weight?
    a. 6 mL
    b. 5 mL
    c. 3 mL
    d. 2.5 mL

12. A patient has been administered 2 g of a drug per 100 mL of solution. This would indicate the patient has received which of the following strength solutions?
    a. 3%
    b. 1%
    c. 2%
    d. 0.5%

13. A patient has just completed a walk down the hospital hallway to determine the oxygen saturation during exercise. The patient walked 1500 cm. How many meters did the patient walk?
    a. 1.5
    b. 5
    c. 15
    d. 20

14. A prescription for an oral medication for a 3-year-old child states to give 1 teaspoon every 8 hours. The mother decides to use a syringe to obtain the medication to give a more exact dosage. How many milliliters of drug should be given?
    a. 1
    b. 3
    c. 5
    d. 6

15. A patient needs 0.5 g of a drug every 8 hours. If each tablet contains a strength of 250 mg, how many tablets should the person take?
    a. 1
    b. 2
    c. 2.5
    d. 1.5

16. A patient in the emergency department (ED) has been ordered to receive Drug A by injection. One ampoule contains 1 mg/mL of Drug A. The order states to give a 0.25-dose subcutaneously. How many milliliters should be administered?
    a. 0.25
    b. 0.50
    c. 1
    d. 1.25

17. A patient admitted for exacerbation of asthma has been ordered to receive albuterol. The order states "albuterol q4h and prn with 5 mg/mL solution by SVN." As you are giving the treatment, the resident making rounds asks what is the percentage strength of the albuterol. Based on the prescription the patient is receiving:
    a. 0.1%
    b. 0.5%
    c. 0.25%
    d. 0.4%

18. The _____ of a drug is the amount of solute in a solution, usually expressed as a percentage.
    a. Solution
    b. Solute
    c. Solvent
    d. Strength

19. On a patient's chart, you read that the patient drank 2 cups of apple juice for breakfast. This would be equal to _____ mL.
    a. 64
    b. 100
    c. 220
    d. 480

20. A 3-mL unit dose of albuterol with a percentage strength of 0.083% is available for administration. What should be done so that the usual dose of 2.5 mg is delivered?
    a. Mix the unit dose with 5 mL of normal saline.
    b. Mix 1 mL of the unit dose and 1 mL of normal saline.
    c. Administer all 3 mL of the unit dose to the patient.
    d. Mix the unit dose with 3 mL of normal saline.

CASE STUDY 1

A resident orders Drug B to be delivered by SVN to one of your patients. The drug is available as 20 mg in 2 mL of aqueous solution. What percentage strength are you delivering to your patient?
(*Hint:* You're doing a weight-to-volume calculation.)

CASE STUDY 2

A 45-year-old patient is admitted to the intensive care unit with Tylenol overdose. The treatment calls for administration of 6 mL of 20% Mucomyst. Only 10% Mucomyst is available. How much 10% Mucomyst is needed to prepare 6 mL of 20% Mucomyst?

CASE STUDY 3

A 6-year-old child is being discharged from the hospital, and the mother has a medication that has a dropper that is able to measure 1 mL. The prescription calls for the child to receive 0.5 mL of the medication every 6 hours. The mother is concerned that she will not get the medication exact.

1. What should the mother do to ensure an exact amount of drug?

The mother states that she has "measuring spoons" that she uses for baking at home, and she feels they are very accurate. She has a one-half teaspoon measuring spoon that she could use to give her child medication, and this way she wouldn't have to count out the drops.

2. What could you say to the mother concerning using household measuring spoons to administer medication?

5 Central and Peripheral Nervous Systems

CHAPTER OUTLINE

Key Terms and Definitions
The Nervous System
    Parasympathetic Branch
    Sympathetic Branch
Cholinergic and Anticholinergic Agents
Neural Control of Lung Function
National Board for Respiratory Care (NBRC) Testing Questions
Case Studies 1 and 2

CHAPTER OBJECTIVES

After answering the following questions, the reader should be able to:

1. Define key terms pertaining to the central and peripheral nervous systems
2. Classify the branches of the nervous system
3. Differentiate among the *central, peripheral,* and *autonomic nervous systems*
4. Discuss the use of *neurotransmitters*
5. Explain in detail the difference between the *parasympathetic* and *sympathetic* branches of the nervous system
6. Differentiate the effects of *cholinergic* and *anticholinergic agents* on the nervous system
7. Differentiate the effects of *adrenergic* and *antiadrenergic agents* on the nervous system
8. Discuss the various receptors in the airways
9. Differentiate among *nonadrenergic, noncholinergic inhibitory,* and *excitatory* nerves

KEY TERMS AND DEFINITIONS

Complete the following questions by writing the correct term in the blanks provided.

1. The portion of the nervous system that includes the brain and spinal cord, controlling voluntary and involuntary acts, is called the _____ _____ _____.

2. The portion of the nervous system that is outside the central nervous system and includes the sensory, sympathetic, and parasympathetic nerves is known as the _____ _____ _____.

3. Signals that are transmitted *from* the brain and spinal cord are called _____.

4. Signals that are transmitted *to* the brain and spinal cord are called _____.

5. The neurotransmitter used at postganglionic sympathetic nerve sites is _____.

6. The neurotransmitter used in the transmission of nerve impulses in the parasympathetic nervous system is _____. It is destroyed by cholinesterase.

7. A drug stimulating a receptor for norepinephrine or epinephrine is called _____.

8. A drug blocking a receptor for acetylcholine is called _____.

9. An agent causing stimulation of parasympathetic nervous system sites is called _____.

10. An agent that blocks the effect of the sympathetic nervous system is called _____.

11. An agent that blocks the effect of the parasympathetic nervous system is called _____.

12. An agent that stimulates the sympathetic nervous system is called _____.

THE NERVOUS SYSTEM

Complete the following questions by writing the correct term in the blank provided.

13. There are two major control systems in the body: the _____ system and the _____ system.

14. The nervous system is divided into two parts. List each part.

    a. _____

    b. _____

15. The parasympathetic and sympathetic nervous systems are contained in the _____ nervous system.

16. The parasympathetic branch arises from the _____ portion of the spinal cord.

17. The sympathetic branch arises from the _____ portion of the spinal cord.

18. Because sympathetic fibers innervate the adrenal medulla, after sympathetic activation there is a release of _____ into the bloodstream.

19. List three characteristics of both the parasympathetic and sympathetic nervous systems.

    Parasympathetic nervous system

    a. _____

    b. _____

    c. _____

    Sympathetic nervous system

    a. _____

    b. _____

    c. _____

20. Give an example of when you need sympathetic nervous system activation.

Note: To understand autonomic drugs, you need to understand neurotransmitters.

21. Neurotransmitters control _____ impulses.

22. The neurotransmitter located in skeletal muscle, the parasympathetic nervous system terminal nerve sites, and all ganglionic synapses is _____.

23. Circle the correct answer: The autonomic nervous system is generally thought to be an (efferent/afferent) system.

24. The neurotransmitter conducting the nerve impulse at smooth muscle sites is _____.

25. Norepinephrine and sympathetic transmission are terminated by _____, _____, and _____.

26. Match each of the following terms with its corresponding definition.

    1. _____ Sympathomimetic
    2. _____ Adrenergic
    3. _____ Parasympatholytic
    4. _____ Anticholinergic
    5. _____ Antiadrenergic
    6. _____ Parasympathomimetic
    7. _____ Cholinergic
    8. _____ Sympatholytic

    a. Agent blocking sympathetic nervous system
    b. Agent stimulating parasympathetic nervous system
    c. Agent blocking epinephrine receptor
    d. Agent blocking acetylcholine receptor
    e. Agent stimulating sympathetic nervous system
    f. Agent stimulating acetylcholine receptor
    g. Agent blocking parasympathetic nervous system
    h. Agent stimulating epinephrine receptor

Parasympathetic Branch

27. Fill in the changes that occur with parasympathetic (cholinergic) stimulation:

    a. Heart: _____
    b. Bronchial smooth muscle: _____
    c. Exocrine glands: _____

28. Two additional terms used to refer to stimulation of receptor sites by acetylcholine are

    a. _____, because of the effect of nicotine, and
    b. _____, because of the effect of muscarine.

29. Circle the correct answer: Administration of a muscarinic drug such as neostigmine (increases/decreases) airway secretions.

30. A parasympathomimetic effect is the same as a _____ effect, and a parasympatholytic effect is the same as a _____ effect.

31. The term *nicotinic* refers to cholinergic receptors on ganglia and at the _____.

CHOLINERGIC AND ANTICHOLINERGIC AGENTS

Complete the following questions by writing the answer in the space provided.

32. Name a direct-acting cholinergic drug that is used to assess the degree of airway reactivity in suspected asthmatic patients: _____

33. An indirect-acting cholinergic agent that is short acting and a useful diagnostic agent for myasthenia gravis is:

    a. Generic name _____

    b. Brand name _____

34. Parasympatholytics and neuromuscular blocking agents block acetylcholine receptors and are therefore _____ agents.

35. An antihistamine drug with an anticholinergic effect, commonly used to prevent motion sickness, is _____.

36. List four uses of a parasympatholytic or antimuscarinic agent such as atropine.

    a. _____

    b. _____

    c. _____

    d. _____

Sympathetic Branch

37. Circle the correct answer: Stimulation of the heart should (increase/decrease) cardiac output.

38. The neurotransmitter at the terminal nerve sites in the sympathetic branch of the autonomic nervous system is _____.

39. The following are sympathomimetic drugs. Fill in their uses.

Drug	Uses
Epinephrine	a. _____
Albuterol	b. _____
Salmeterol	c. _____
Dopamine	d. _____

40. List two types of sympathetic receptors.

    a. _____

    b. _____

41. Stimulation of alpha (α) receptors causes _____.

42. Stimulation of beta$_1$ (β_1) receptors increases the _____ and _____ _____ of cardiac smooth muscle.

43. Stimulation of β_{12} receptors causes _____ and _____ muscle relaxation.

44. Which receptors (α, β_{11}, or β_{12}) would be best to stimulate if a patient had a runny nose?

45. Which receptors (α, β_{11}, or β_{11}) would be best to stimulate to give relief to a patient in the midst of an asthma attack?

46. The chemical found in the brain that is a precursor of norepinephrine and stimulates both α and β receptors is called _____.

NEURAL CONTROL OF LUNG FUNCTION

Complete the following questions by writing the correct term in the blank provided.

47. Although no direct sympathetic innervation of airway smooth muscle occurs, the sympathetic nervous system controls smooth muscle tone by circulating _____.

48. Epinephrine acts on both _____ and _____ receptors, whereas norepinephrine acts primarily on _____ receptors.

49. β Agonists, distributed from the trachea to terminal bronchioles, cause _____ of small airways.

50. True or False: Adrenergic receptors in the lung are all β_2 receptors.

51. True or False: β_1 receptors are located in the alveolar walls and lung periphery.

52. True or False: The α receptors are located equally throughout large and small airways and are less abundant than β receptors.

53. The lung receives its blood supply from both the _____ and the _____ circulations.

54. Pulmonary circulation is innervated by both the _____ _____ _____ and the _____ _____ nervous systems.

55. Arterial (bronchial) circulation is innervated mostly by the _____ _____ _____.

56. Bronchial submucosal glands are innervated by the _____ _____ _____ and _____ _____ _____.

57. True or False. When bronchial mucosal glands are stimulated, less mucus is produced.

58. Airway smooth muscle responds to circulating _____ by means of β receptors.

59. Submucosal glands have both _____ and _____ receptors.

60. The lung is innervated by the _____ nerve, which enters the lung at the hilum and innervates intrapulmonary airways.

61. Stimulation of the vagus nerve as it relates to the bronchial smooth muscle causes _____.

62. Circle the correct answer: Stimulation of the vagus nerve causes submucosal glands to (increase/decrease) secretions.

63. Three muscarinic receptor sites are present in the lung. Which of these, M_1, M_2, or M_3, is located on submucosal glands and airway smooth muscle? _____

64. Muscarinic receptor M_3 is located on blood vessels and causes the release of an endothelial-derived relaxant factor that produces _____ of the both bronchial and pulmonary vasculature.

65. Evidence indicates a branch of nerves other than adrenergic or cholinergic that cause bronchodilation. These nerves are called _____ and _____ system.

66. Inhibitory effects on airway smooth muscle cause bronchodilation and may be mediated by the neurotransmitter _____ or by _____ _____.

67. Excitatory effects such as bronchoconstriction are produced by afferent sensory fibers that have _____ _____ as a neurotransmitter.

NATIONAL BOARD FOR RESPIRATORY CARE (NBRC) TESTING QUESTIONS

1. The sympathetic nervous system is part of which of the following?
   a. Central nervous system
   b. Peripheral nervous system
   c. Autonomic nervous system
   d. Both b and c

2. Which branch of the nervous system controls daily functions, such as digestion and bladder control?
   a. Central nervous system
   b. Parasympathetic nervous system
   c. Sympathetic nervous system
   d. Both b and c

3. Which of the following describes a drug that stimulates the sympathetic nervous system?
   a. Parasympathomimetic
   b. Parasympatholytic
   c. Sympathomimetic
   d. Sympatholytic

4. Which of the following describes the autonomic nervous system?
   a. Sends impulses from the brain to the neuroeffector sites (e.g., heart and lungs)
   b. Sends impulses from the periphery to the brain and spinal cord
   c. Is exemplified by the knee-jerk reaction
   d. Is an afferent system

5. Which of the following describes a drug that blocks a receptor for acetylcholine?
   a. Cholinergic
   b. Anticholinergic
   c. Adrenergic
   d. Antiadrenergic

6. Sympathetic nervous system stimulation results in which of the following?
   a. Decreased blood pressure
   b. Mental stimulation
   c. Decreased heart rate
   d. Bronchoconstriction

7. Which two enzymes inactivate catecholamines?
   a. TDH and BHG
   b. COTN and MNM
   c. AchE and TKO
   d. COMT and MAO

8. Stimulation of which of the following receptors results in vasoconstriction?
   a. α
   b. β_1
   c. β_2
   d. γ

9. Epinephrine accomplishes which of the following?
   a. Stimulates primarily α receptors
   b. Stimulates primarily β receptors
   c. Stimulates α and β receptors equally
   d. Stimulates neither α nor β receptors

10. Blood flow to the lung is supplied by which of the following?
    1. Pulmonary circulation
    2. Vagal circulation
    3. Bronchial circulation
    4. Parasympathetic circulation
       a. 1 and 4 only
       b. 2 and 3 only
       c. 1 and 3 only
       d. 2 and 4 only

11. Bronchodilation most likely occurs as a result of stimulation of which receptor?
    a. α_1
    b. α_2
    c. β_1
    d. β_2

12. Relaxation of airway smooth muscle should *not* occur with which of the following?
    a. Stimulation of the nonadrenergic inhibitory nerves
    b. Use of a cholinergic agent
    c. Use of a sympathomimetic
    d. Use of a parasympatholytic

13. A drug that stimulates the parasympathetic nervous system will cause which of the following?
    a. Slower heart rate
    b. Bronchodilation
    c. Reduced secretions
    d. Thicker secretions

14. Which of the following are sympathomimetic or adrenergic agonists?
    1. Epinephrine
    2. Propranolol
    3. Albuterol
    4. Salmeterol
       a. 1 and 4 only
       b. 1, 2 and 3 only
       c. 1, 3 and 4 only
       d. 1, 2, 3 and 4

15. Adrenergic receptors in the lung are:
    a. All α_1
    b. All β_1
    c. All β_2
    d. α_1 and β_2

16. Bronchial submucosal glands are innervated by:
    a. Parasympathetic nervous system
    b. Sympathetic nervous system
    c. Both parasympathetic and sympathetic nervous systems
    d. Central nervous system

17. The nerve that innervates the lung and enters at the hilum is the:
    a. Phrenic
    b. Pulmonic
    c. Glossopharyngeal
    d. Vagus

18. Stimulation of β_1 receptors of cardiac smooth muscle will cause which of the following?
    1. Increased heart rate
    2. Reduced cardiac output
    3. Coronary artery constriction
    4. Increased force of contraction
       a. 1 and 3 only
       b. 1 and 4 only
       c. 1, 2, and 3 only
       d. 1, 2, 3, and 4

19. A patient has just received a medication and is now experiencing relief from an exacerbation of asthma. Based on this information, which of the following agonists was given?
    a. α_1
    b. β_1
    c. α_2
    d. β_2

20. Which of the following would be a sympathomimetic effect of epinephrine?
    a. Bronchodilation
    b. Miosis
    c. Vasodilation
    d. Bradycardia

21. A direct-acting cholinergic agent used to help diagnose asthma is:
    a. Mestinon
    b. Methacholine
    c. Pilocarpine
    d. Tensilon

22. Which of the following drugs is a muscarinic that increases airway secretions?
    a. Neostigmine
    b. Epinephrine
    c. Atropine
    d. Albuterol

23. To help reduce airway secretions during surgery, which of the following drugs is given before surgery in patients?
    a. Tensilon
    b. Epinephrine
    c. Atropine
    d. Pilocarpine

24. Which of the following muscarinic receptor sites found in the lung is located on submucosal glands and smooth muscle?
    a. M_1
    b. M_2
    c. M_3
    d. M_5

25. To relieve nasal congestion, you would purchase a medication that has which of the following drug ingredients?
    a. Ephedrine
    b. Amphetamine
    c. Albuterol
    d. Salmeterol

CASE STUDY 1

Methacholine is an inhaled parasympathomimetic agent used in bronchial challenge tests to determine the degree of airway reactivity in asthmatic individuals.

1. What is the parasympathetic effect?

2. Explain how methacholine works to detect the degree of airway reactivity?

CASE STUDY 2

A 49-year-old woman has entered the emergency department (ED) with complaints of weakness involving her face, eyes, and arms. The patient explains that she has experienced blurred vision that comes and goes, and also her eyelids are drooping. She further states that she has problems swallowing, and she sometimes chokes when swallowing liquids. Additionally, she notes that recently she has had difficulty lifting light objects. After the ED doctor consults with a neurologist, it is concluded that she may have myasthenia gravis, and the decision is made to do an edrophonium (Tensilon) test.

1. What is the purpose of administering edrophonium (Tensilon) this patient?

2. Why is this drug classified as an indirect-acting cholinergic agonist?

3. Why is edrophonium used?

4. Tensilon can be administered by two routes, either pill or intravenously. Which would be the best route of administration for this patient? Explain your answer.

5. What indirect-acting cholinergic maintenance drug is prescribed for muscle stimulation for patients with myasthenia gravis?

6. What are two undesirable effects associated with the use of either of these indirect cholinergic maintenance drugs?
   a. _____
   b. _____

UNIT TWO DRUGS USED TO TREAT THE RESPIRATORY SYSTEM

6 Adrenergic (Sympathomimetic) Bronchodilators

CHAPTER OUTLINE

Key Terms and Definitions
Clinical Indications for Adrenergic Bronchodilators
Long-Acting β-Adrenergic Agents
Mode of Action
Routes of Administration
Adverse Side Effects
β-Agonist Controversy
Respiratory Care Assessment of β-Agonist Therapy
National Board of Respiratory Care (NBRC) Testing Questions
Case Studies 1 and 2

CHAPTER OBJECTIVES

After answering the following questions, the reader should be able to:

1. Define terms that pertain to drugs used to treat the respiratory system
2. List all currently available β-adrenergic agents used in respiratory therapy
3. Differentiate between the specific adrenergic agents and formulations
4. Describe the mechanism of action for each specific adrenergic agent and formulation
5. Describe the route of administration available for β agonists
6. Discuss adverse effects of β agonists
7. Clinically assess β-agonist therapy

Chapter 6 is of particular importance because inhaled adrenergic bronchodilators represent the drugs most commonly administered by respiratory therapists.

KEY TERMS AND DEFINITIONS

Complete the following questions by writing the correct answer in the blank provided.

1. An enzyme that produces a reaction the opposite of that of cyclic adenosine monophosphate (cAMP), and causes bronchoconstriction, is _____.

2. A _____ produces effects similar to those of the sympathetic nervous system.

3. Narrowing of the airways resulting from contraction of smooth muscle is called _____.

4. A group of similar compounds having sympathomimetic action and mimicking the actions of epinephrine is the _____.

5. An agent that stimulates sympathetic nervous fibers and allows relaxation of smooth muscle in the airway is a _____ _____.

6. A drug that exhibits pharmacologic activity once it is converted, inside the body, to its active form, is called a _____.

7. _____ stimulation causes vasoconstriction and a vasopressor effect in the upper airway, which provides decongestion.

8. _____ stimulation causes increased myocardial conductivity, heart rate, and contractile force.

9. Long-term desensitization of β receptors to $β_2$ agonists, caused by a reduction in the number of β receptors, is called _____.

10. _____ stimulation causes relaxation of bronchial smooth muscle with some inhibition of inflammatory mediator release and stimulation of mucociliary clearance.

11. _____ _____ refers to the increasing incidence of asthma morbidity, and especially asthma mortality, despite advances in the understanding of asthma and availability of improved drugs to treat asthma.

12. _____ _____ is a nucleotide-produced $β_2$-receptor stimulation that causes relaxation of bronchial smooth muscle.

13. What are the results of α and $β_1$ receptor stimulation?

14. List three effects that $β_2$-specific drugs produce.

    a. _____

    b. _____

    c. _____

CLINICAL INDICATIONS FOR ADRENERGIC BRONCHODILATORS

15. What is the general indication for adrenergic bronchodilators?

16. List three short-acting adrenergic bronchodilators.

    a. _____

    b. _____

    c. _____

17. List five long-acting adrenergic bronchodilators.

    a. _____

    b. _____

    c. _____

    d. _____

    e. _____

18. What is the major difference between the indication for short-acting agents compared with long-acting agents?

19. Please take the time to visit the following websites:
    http://www.nhlbi.nih.gov/health-pro/guidelines/current/asthma-guidelines
    http://www.ginasthma.org

20. List three indications for administration of racemic epinephrine.

    a. _____

    b. _____

    c. _____

21. Put a check mark next to the symptom(s) that occur(s) with administration of a catecholamine:

    a. Tachycardia: _____

    b. Bronchoconstriction: _____

    c. Elevated blood pressure: _____

    d. Bronchodilation: _____

    e. Increased urine output: _____

    f. Relaxation of skeletal muscle blood vessels: _____

22. Why shouldn't catecholamines be given orally?

23. What enzyme metabolizes epinephrine?

24. Explain how catecholamines were made more β_2 specific.

25. List four ways in which albuterol can be delivered.

    a. _____

    b. _____

    c. _____

    d. _____

26. List three trade names for albuterol that a respiratory therapist can deliver via inhalation.

    a. _____

    b. _____

    c. _____

27. What is a prodrug?

28. List the three strengths of nebulized solutions of levalbuterol that are available.

    a. _____

    b. _____

    c. _____

29. The brand name for levalbuterol is _____.

30. List eight effects and characteristics of the (S)-isomer of albuterol.

    a. _____

    b. _____

    c. _____

    d. _____

    e. _____

    f. _____

    g. _____

    h. _____

31. Fill in the blanks regarding levalbuterol (Xopenex):

    a. Onset of action: _____

    b. Peak effect: _____

    c. Duration of effect: _____

    d. Receptor preference: _____

    e. Routes available: _____

LONG-ACTING β-ADRENERGIC AGENTS

32. Fill in the chart regarding long-acting bronchodilator agents.

Generic Name	Brand Name	Receptor Preference	Adult Dosage	Time Course (Onset, Peak, Duration)
Salmeterol				
Formoterol				
Arformoterol				
Indacterol				
Olodaterol				

33. VoSpire ER is an extended-release form of _____ that has an extended activity up to _____ hours.

34. List four points that should be noted in the clinical use of long-acting agents because of their differences from shorter-acting β agonists.

    a.

    b.

    c.

d.

35. Because of the ongoing safety concerns regarding long-acting β_2 agonists, the U.S. Food and Drug Administration (FDA) is now requiring changes on how long-acting β_2 agonists are used in the treatment of asthma. List five of these requirements.

   a.

   b.

   c.

   d.

   e.

36. *Circle True or False in the following statements:*
   a. True or False: National guidelines recommend the introduction of a long-acting β agonist in asthma requiring step 3 care; it should be used as deemed necessary for chronic obstructive pulmonary disease (COPD).
   b. True or False: Use of long-acting β agonists may prevent the need to increase the inhaled dose of corticosteroid.

c. True or False: Long-acting β_2 agonists are recommended for rescue bronchodilation.
d. True or False: Asthmatic patients must be educated in the use of both short-acting and long-acting bronchodilators.
e. True or False: Both the short-acting and long-acting β_2 agonists can be substituted for inhaled corticosteroids because of their antiinflammatory effects.
f. True or False: The Advair Diskus inhaler is a combination product of both salmeterol and fluticasone that has demonstrated superior asthma control and better lung function than either drug taken alone.

MODE OF ACTION

37. Match the following modes of action with the type of receptor stimulation:
    1. _____ Upper airway vasoconstriction
    2. _____ Relaxation of bronchial smooth muscle
    3. _____ Stimulation of mucociliary clearance
    4. _____ Increased heart rate
    5. _____ Decongestion in the nasal passages
    6. _____ Increased contractile force of the heart
    7. _____ Some inhibition of inflammatory mediator release

    a. α-Receptor stimulation
    b. β_1-Receptor stimulation
    c. β_2-Receptor stimulation

ROUTES OF ADMINISTRATION

38. The following is a list of routes of administration. Indicate for each route whether it is currently available *(Y for Yes)* or not available *(N for No)* for β-adrenergic bronchodilators:
    a. metered dose inhaler (MDI): _____
    b. dry powder inhaler (DPI): _____
    c. Tablet: _____
    d. Syrup: _____
    e. Nebulizer solution: _____
    f. Parenteral: _____
    g. Suppository: _____

39. List five reasons why inhalation is the preferred route of administration of a β-adrenergic drug:
    a. _____
    b. _____
    c. _____
    d. _____
    e. _____

40. Why must catecholamines be given via inhalation?

41. List five advantages of the oral inhalation route in administering β agonists.

    a. _____

    b. _____

    c. _____

    d. _____

    e. _____

ADVERSE SIDE EFFECTS

42. Adverse side effects can occur with β agonists. Name three side effects.

    a. _____

    b. _____

    c. _____

43. What does *tolerance* mean?

44. A fall in the partial pressure of arterial oxygen (Pa_{O_2}) has been noted with newer β agonists, such as albuterol and salmeterol. Explain why.

β-AGONIST CONTROVERSY

45. Despite our increased understanding of asthma and the availability of improved drug treatment, asthma morbidity and mortality seem to be increasing. The role that $β_2$ drugs play in this phenomenon is unclear. List five possible reasons suggested by the literature.

    a.

    b.

c.

d.

e.

RESPIRATORY CARE ASSESSMENT OF β-AGONIST THERAPY

46. *Circle True or False in the following statements:*
    a. True or False: A peak flow meter can be used to assess the reversibility of airflow obstruction at the bedside.
    b. True or False: The respiratory care practitioner should assess breathing rate and pattern and breath sounds before and after the completion of treatment.
    c. True or False: Potassium can decrease and blood glucose can increase with the use of continuous nebulization of a β agonist.
    d. True or False: When educating a patient about asthma, it should be emphasized that only β agonists are needed to prevent severe asthma episodes.
    e. True or False: Patient education should include the correct use of aerosol devices, as well as assembly and cleaning of devices.
    f. True or False: When assessing a patient to determine the benefit of long-acting β agonists, the respiratory care practitioner should assess nocturnal symptoms, number of exacerbations, unscheduled clinic or hospital visits, and days of absence from work related to symptoms.

NATIONAL BOARD OF RESPIRATORY CARE (NBRC) TESTING QUESTIONS

1. $β_2$-Receptor stimulation has which of the following effects?
   a. Mucous gland hypertrophy
   b. Bronchial smooth muscle relaxation
   c. Decreased peripheral blood flow
   d. Increased pulmonary blood flow

2. Catecholamines do which of the following?
   a. Mimic the action of catechol
   b. Mimic the action of epinephrine
   c. Have a prolamine nucleus
   d. Are α inhibitors

3. Which of the following describes catecholamines?
   a. Long acting
   b. Slow onset
   c. Useful for asthma maintenance therapy
   d. Inactivated by catechol-*O*-methyltransferase (COMT)

4. Catecholamines are unsuitable for which route of administration?
   a. Intravenous
   b. Inhalation
   c. Oral
   d. Subcutaneous

5. Metaproterenol is an example of which type of adrenergic bronchodilator?
   a. Catecholamine
   b. Resorcinol
   c. Saligenin
   d. Sustained release

6. Which of the following drugs is a long-acting bronchodilator?
   a. Terbutaline
   b. Epinephrine
   c. Indacterol
   d. Proventil

7. Which of the following strengths are available for nebulization of levalbuterol?
   1. 0.31 mg
   2. 0.63 mg
   3. 1.25 mg
   4. 2.50 mg
      a. 1 and 2 only
      b. 2 and 4 only
      c. 1, 2, and 3 only
      d. 1, 2, 3, and 4

8. Perforomist can be given as a liquid nebulization and is approved only for:
   a. Exercise-induced asthma
   b. Asthma with nocturnal sleeping problems
   c. COPD
   d. Pulmonary fibrosis

9. Which of the following catecholamines or catecholamine derivatives lasts the longest?
   a. Albuterol
   b. Racemic epinephrine
   c. Metaproterenol
   d. Salmeterol

10. All but which of the following diseases is likely to respond well to adrenergic bronchodilators?
    a. Asthma
    b. Cystic fibrosis
    c. Chronic bronchitis
    d. Pulmonary fibrosis

11. Which of the following drugs can be administered both subcutaneously and by inhalation to treat asthma exacerbation?
    a. Acetylcholine
    b. Norepinephrine
    c. Epinephrine
    d. Dopamine

12. Which of the following is a form of single-isomer albuterol?
    a. Salmeterol
    b. Levalbuterol
    c. Terbutaline
    d. Asthmanefrin

13. In relation to bronchodilators, "rescue" agents refer to:
    a. Short-acting agents
    b. Long-acting agents
    c. Controllers
    d. Prodrugs

14. Which of the following are saligenins?
    1. Terbutaline
    2. Epinephrine
    3. Levalbuterol
    4. Albuterol
        a. 1 and 2 only
        b. 3 and 4 only
        c. 1, 2, and 3 only
        d. 1, 2, 3, and 4

15. Which of the following are short-acting bronchodilators?
    1. Albuterol
    2. Metaproterenol
    3. Levalbuterol
    4. Salmeterol
        a. 1 and 3 only
        b. 1, 3, and 4 only
        c. 1, 2, and 3 only
        d. 1, 2, 3, and 4

16. What strength of racemic epinephrine is used for nebulization?
    a. 2.25%
    b. 1%
    c. 3%
    d. 1.25%

17. Albuterol is available in a variety of pharmaceutical vehicles, including:
    1. Tablets
    2. Syrup
    3. Nebulizer solution
    4. MDI
        a. 1 and 3 only
        b. 2 and 3 only
        c. 2, 3, and 4 only
        d. 1, 2, 3, and 4

18. Which of the following are side effects associated with β agonists?
    1. Tremor
    2. Palpitations
    3. Tachycardia
    4. Headache
        a. 1 and 2 only
        b. 2 and 4 only
        c. 2, 3, and 4 only
        d. 1, 2, 3, and 4

19. Exposure to which of the following readily inactivates catecholamines?
    a. Oxygen
    b. Saline
    c. Light
    d. Air

20. The only pure (R)-isomer of racemic albuterol that is a short-acting bronchodilator available in the U.S. market is:
    a. Xopenex
    b. Severent
    c. Tornalate
    d. Maxair

21. Formoterol, like salmeterol, has a long-lasting bronchodilating effect up to _____ hours of duration.
    a. 6
    b. 5
    c. 12
    d. 23

22. Aformoterol is a long-acting $β_2$-selective agonist that is approved by the FDA as:
    a. Stovana
    b. Afrobrovana
    c. Brovona
    d. R-Stovana

23. National guidelines recommend the introduction of a long-acting β agonist in step 3 care of asthma when which of the following conditions exists?
    a. Asthma controlled by short-acting β agonists
    b. Asthma not controlled by lower doses of antiinflammatory medicine
    c. Asthma not controlled by higher doses of antiinflammatory medicine
    d. Asthma not controlled by short-acting β agonist and high doses of antiinflammatory medicine

24. Which of the following statements regarding the drop in Pa_{O_2} after bronchodilator administration by inhalation is true?
    1. It occurs because of ventilation-perfusion mismatch.
    2. The drop is physiologically significant.
    3. The drop is statistically significant.
    4. The drop in oxygen saturation (Sa_{O_2}) is minimal.
        a. 2 only
        b. 1 and 3 only
        c. 1, 3, and 4 only
        d. 2, 3, and 4 only

25. The general indication for adrenergic bronchodilators is to:
    a. Reduce the consistency of mucus
    b. Reduce inflammation
    c. Reduce blood flow to target organs
    d. Reverse or lessen the degree of airflow obstruction

26. Epinephrine is a potent catecholamine bronchodilator; in addition, what other receptors does it effect?
    a. α only
    b. β_1 only
    c. α and β_1
    d. β_2 only

27. A pediatric patient has stridor and has been diagnosed with croup. To help reduce the swelling in the upper airway, which drug would be most beneficial?
    a. Racemic epinephrine
    b. Terbutaline
    c. Albuterol
    d. Levalbuterol

28. Albuterol has which of the following actions?
    1. Duration up to 5 to 8 hours
    2. β_2 preferential
    3. Peak effect within 30 to 60 minutes
    4. Can be delivered by mouth
    a. 1 and 2 only
    b. 2 and 3 only
    c. 1, 2, and 3 only
    d. 1, 2, 3, and 4

29. This drug is used for prevention of acute exercise-induced bronchospasm in adults and children older than 5 years of age:
    a. Salmeterol
    b. Levalbuterol
    c. Albuterol
    d. Formoterol

30. The National Asthma Education and Prevention Program (NAEPP) Expert Panel Report 3 (EPR 3) Guidelines on Asthma consider salmeterol to be which of the following types of drug?
    a. Controller
    b. Rescue
    c. Reliever
    d. Short term and rescue

31. Asthmatic patients must be educated that the use of β agonists will:
    a. Treat inflammation
    b. Treat poor pulmonary blood flow
    c. Be used as a rescue medication for exacerbations of their asthma
    d. Prevent the use of medication to treat aggressive asthma

32. Which of the following is a reason why inhalation is the preferred route of administration of a β-adrenergic drug?
    a. Slow onset
    b. Larger dose required compared with the oral route
    c. Reduced side effects
    d. Reduced lung availability/total systemic availability (L/T) ratio

33. A practical approach to optimal drug dosing in a patient brought to the emergency department with severe airway obstruction, and who does not respond to intermittent nebulizer treatments after 1 hour, would be _____ _____ of β agonists.
    a. Increasing dosage
    b. Oral administration
    c. Subcutaneous injection
    d. Continuous nebulization

34. A respiratory therapist tells the physician that he is measuring the bronchodilating effect of a β agonist. The therapist would be:
    a. Determining the reaction of the airway by cold air introduction
    b. Determining the reaction of the airway by the amount of wheezing produced by methacholine challenge
    c. Measuring airflow changes by measuring forced expiratory volume at 1 second (FEV_1)
    d. Determining the reaction of the airway by introduction of histamine

35. Which of the following would be used to assess reversibility of airflow obstruction?
    1. Peak flow meter
    2. Incentive spirometer
    3. Portable spirometry
    4. Pulse oximetry
        a. 1 and 3 only
        b. 2 and 4 only
        c. 1, 3, and 4 only
        d. 2, 3, and 4 only

36. To assess the effectiveness of long-acting β agonists, you would do which of the following?
    a. Assess ongoing lung function by peak expiratory flow
    b. Send patient questionnaire every 6 weeks
    c. Obtain blood culture every 6 months
    d. Assess ongoing lung function by serial radiologic studies

37. Which of the following should be assessed to determine the benefit of long-acting β agonists in an asthmatic patient?
    1. Nocturnal symptoms
    2. Number of exacerbations
    3. Unscheduled clinic or hospital visits
    4. Days of absence from work related to symptoms
        a. 1 and 2 only
        b. 2 and 3 only
        c. 1, 2, and 4 only
        d. 1, 2, 3, and 4

38. To manage severe asthma and avoid respiratory failure, intubation, and mechanical ventilation, which of the following methods of administration of inhaled adrenergic bronchodilation is recommended by the NAEPP EPR 3 guidelines?
    a. Small volume nebulizer every 10 minutes × 5 times
    b. Small volume nebulizer every 60 minutes × 3 times
    c. MDI, 12 to 20 puffs every 4 hours
    d. Continuous nebulizer, 10 to 15 mg/hr

39. Children being treated for asthma should use only which of the following in conjunction with a corticosteroid?
    a. Short-acting agonist
    b. Long-acting agonist
    c. α_1 Stimulator
    d. Catecholamine

40. The extended-release form of albuterol, VoSpire ER, is delivered in which of the following ways?
    a. Tablet
    b. pressurized MDI (pMDI)
    c. Breath-actuated MDI
    d. Liquid

CASE STUDY 1

A 16-year-old patient suffers from moderate asthma. He is receiving a regimen of cromolyn sodium and corticosteroid.

1. What would be the best choice of sympathomimetic bronchodilator to accompany this therapy?

2. What is the one condition in which the sympathomimetic bronchodilator you chose in question 1 would be likely to cause your patient problems?

CASE STUDY 2

You are an asthma educator working in a doctor's office. Candace is 27-year-old woman who has been diagnosed with asthma. She is ordered to receive a β_2 agonist by pMDI. You and the doctor are meeting with her to review her medications and answer any questions Candace may have at this time. After some discussion, the doctor leaves, but Candace would like the educator to answer more of her questions concerning her drugs.

1. Candace would like to know why she has to take this drug by inhalation instead of taking it by tablet or syrup.

2. Candace says she knows the drug helps her airways "open up," but asks whether there is any other way she could see whether her drug is working.

3. Candace would also like to know whether this drug has side effects.

4. Candace is concerned about the drug's effect on her heart. What can the educator tell her to do to monitor for this effect, and when should she be concerned about her heart rate?

5. Candace asks: "What if the β_2 agonist doesn't control my asthma? Is there another medication that I can take?"

7 Anticholinergic (Parasympatholytic) Bronchodilators

CHAPTER OUTLINE

Key Terms and Definitions
Clinical Indications for Use
Specific Anticholinergic (Parasympatholytic) Agents
Pharmacologic Effects of Anticholinergic (Antimuscarinic) Agents
Mode of Action
    Vagally Mediated Reflex Bronchospasm
Clinical Application
    Use in Chronic Obstructive Pulmonary Disease
    Use in Asthma
Combination Therapy: β-Adrenergic Plus Anticholinergic Agents
Respiratory Care Assessment of Anticholinergic Bronchodilator Therapy
National Board of Respiratory Care (NBRC) Testing Questions
Case Studies 1 and 2

CHAPTER OBJECTIVES

After answering the following questions, the reader should be able to:

1. Define terms that pertain to anticholinergic bronchodilators
2. Differentiate between *parasympathomimetic* and *parasympatholytic*
3. Differentiate between *cholinergic* and *anticholinergic*
4. Differentiate between *muscarinic* and *antimuscarinic*
5. List all available anticholinergic agents used in respiratory therapy
6. Discuss the indication for anticholinergic agents
7. Explain the mode of action for anticholinergic agents
8. Identify the routes of administration available for anticholinergic agents
9. Discuss adverse effects for anticholinergic agents
10. Discuss the clinical application for anticholinergic agents

KEY TERMS AND DEFINITIONS

Complete the following questions by writing the answer in the space provided.

1. An agent that blocks parasympathetic nervous fibers is called _____.

2. An agent that produces the effect of acetylcholine is called _____.

3. An agent that blocks parasympathetic nervous fibers, which allow relaxation of smooth muscle in the airway, is called a(n) _____ _____.

4. _____ is the same as *cholinergic*, producing the effect of acetylcholine or an agent that mimics acetylcholine.

5. The word _____ has the same meaning as *anticholinergic*: blocking the effect of acetylcholine at the cholinergic site.

6. A _____ agent produces effects similar to those of the parasympathetic nervous system.

CLINICAL INDICATIONS FOR USE

Complete the following questions by writing the correct term in the blank provided.

7. List four anticholinergic bronchodilators that are indicated as a bronchodilator for maintenance and treatment in chronic obstructive pulmonary disease (COPD), including chronic bronchitis and emphysema (give generic names).

    a. _____
    b. _____
    c. _____
    d. _____

8. A combination of an _____ with a _____ is indicated for use in patients needing regular treatment for COPD and who require additional bronchodilation for relief of airflow obstruction.

9. What two medications make up Combivent?

    a. _____
    b. _____

10. The combination of umeclidinium and vilanterol is called _____ _____.

11. The medication commonly used in severe asthma, especially bronchoconstriction that does not respond well to β-agonist therapy, is _____.

SPECIFIC ANTICHOLINERGIC (PARASYMPATHOLYTIC) AGENTS

Complete the following questions by writing the correct term in the blank provided.

12. List the brand names for the following.

    a. Tiotropium bromide: _____
    b. Ipratropium bromide: _____
    c. Ipratropium bromide and albuterol (metered dose inhaler [MDI]): _____
    d. Ipratropium bromide and albuterol (small volume nebulizer [SVN]): _____
    e. Aclidinium bromide: _____
    f. Umeclidinium bromide: _____

Match the administration method to the correct drug. (Some may require more than one answer.)

13. _____ MDI
14. _____ Soft-mist inhaler
15. _____ SVN
16. _____ Dry powder inhaler (DPI)

a. Atrovent
b. Combivent
c. DuoNeb
d. Spiriva
e. Incruse Ellipta
f. Tudorza Pressair
g. Combivent Respimat

17. Complete the following table for inhaled anticholinergic bronchodilator agents.

Drug	Brand Name	Adult Dosage	Time Course (Onset, Peak, Duration)
Ipatropium bromide			
Ipratropium bromide and albuterol			
Aclidinium bromide			
Tiotropium bromide			
Umeclidinium bromide			
Umeclidinium bromide and vilanterol			

18. Ipratropium bromide is a derivative of _____ _____.

19. Atropine is a _____ _____ _____ and not fully ionized; it therefore is readily absorbed into the bloodstream, is distributed throughout the body, crosses the blood-brain barrier, and causes changes in the central nervous system (CNS).

20. Explain how the clinical effect for ipratropium differs from that for albuterol.

21. Explain the receptor selectivity of tiotropium bromide. How does this explain once-a-day dosing?

22. Your patient has recently been prescribed umeclidinium bromide by his primary care physician and needs an explanation of how it works. What would you tell him?

23. What pharmacologic effects do ipratropium and tiotropium have on the respiratory and cardiac systems?

PHARMACOLOGIC EFFECTS OF ANTICHOLINERGIC (ANTIMUSCARINIC) AGENTS

24. Your patient has just received an inappropriately high dose of atropine. Explain the pharmacologic effects you would expect to see during a physical assessment.

MODE OF ACTION

25. Parasympathetic neurons from what cranial nerve enter the lung at the hila and travel along the airways?

26. Explain why the administration of an anticholinergic can cause significant bronchodilation.

Complete the following questions by writing the correct term in the blank provided.

27. Explain why methacholine is used in bronchial provocation testing.

28. The anticholinergic agents ipratropium and tiotropium are indicated for the treatment of _____ _____ in COPD.

Vagally Mediated Reflex Bronchospasm

29. When sensory C-fiber nerves are stimulated, what clinical manifestation may the patient present with?

30. List the two most common side effects seen with the anticholinergic aerosol ipratropium.

   a. _____

   b. _____

The following questions concern delivery of a quaternary ammonium antimuscarinic bronchodilator, such as ipratropium bromide. Identify each statement as either true or false.

31. True or False: The nebulized dose of ipratropium is more than 10 times greater than the MDI dose, which causes greater systemic effects.

32. True or False: Patients should use a holding chamber with MDI administration.

33. True or False: With nebulizer delivery, the patient must be instructed to keep the mouthpiece in the mouth, and a reservoir tube should be attached to the expiratory side of the T mouthpiece facing away from the patient.

34. True or False: Face mask delivery is recommended to deliver the maximal dose of the drug.

CLINICAL APPLICATION

35. Complete the following table by comparing the general clinical effects of anticholinergic and β-adrenergic bronchodilators.

	Anticholinergic	β Agonist
a. Onset		
b. Time to peak effect		
c. Duration		
d. Fall in arterial partial pressure of oxygen (Pa_{O_2})		
e. Site of action		

Use in Chronic Obstructive Pulmonary Disease

36. Where in the airway do anticholinergic bronchodilators seem to have their greatest effect?

37. The U.S. Food and Drug Administration (FDA) has given approval for ipratropium specifically for use in the treatment of _____, and the drug can also be prescribed for the treatment of _____.

Use in Asthma

38. Besides improving lung function in COPD and controlling symptoms, tiotropium may also be useful for controlling _____ _____ symptoms and deterioration of flow rates at nighttime.

39. Anticholinergics may be useful in patients with acute severe episodes of asthma not responding to _____.

COMBINATION THERAPY: β-ADRENERGIC PLUS ANTICHOLINERGIC AGENTS

40. Anticholinergics act primarily on the _____ airways; β agonists act primarily on the _____ airways.

41. True or False: Because albuterol peaks sooner and terminates sooner, and ipratropium peaks slowly and lasts longer, they complement each other.

42. Combined _____ and _____ therapy may give additive bronchodilating results in COPD and in severe, acute asthma.

43. True or False: An anticholinergic bronchodilator, because of its action on central large airways, should be given before a β agonist.

44. Long-term agents that help reduce the progression of COPD and improve lung function have been termed *triple therapy*. Name the three agents that fall into this category.

    a. _____

    b. _____

    c. _____

RESPIRATORY CARE ASSESSMENT OF ANTICHOLINERGIC BRONCHODILATOR THERAPY

45. List four respiratory care assessments you should perform before the delivery of anticholinergic bronchodilator therapy.

    a. _____

    b. _____

    c. _____

    d. _____

46. List two respiratory care assessments you should perform during the delivery of anticholinergic bronchodilator therapy.

    a. _____

    b. _____

47. List five respiratory care assessments you should perform after the delivery of and for long-term use of anticholinergic bronchodilator therapy.

   a. _____

   b. _____

   c. _____

   d. _____

   e. _____

NATIONAL BOARD OF RESPIRATORY CARE (NBRC) TESTING QUESTIONS

1. An agent that blocks parasympathetic nervous fibers, which allow relaxation of airway smooth muscle, is called:
   a. A parasympathomimetic
   b. An anticholinergic
   c. A muscarinic
   d. A cholinergic

2. A physician has written an order to give a patient Combivent; the order provides no other information. How many puffs and how often should the patient receive this treatment?
   a. Two puffs, qid
   b. Two puffs, qd
   c. Two puffs, bid
   d. Two puffs, q4h

3. A patient calls the pulmonary rehabilitation department and tells the therapist that she has been taking Incruse Ellipta twice per day for the past 2 days. The respiratory therapist should tell the patient to:
   a. Continue on this routine
   b. Increase the treatment to three times per day
   c. Take the medication once per day
   d. Increase the treatment to four times per day

4. The total dose of Atrovent HFA in one puff is:
   a. 17 µg
   b. 34 µg
   c. 39 µg
   d. 100 µg

5. A drug with cholinergic effects would result in which of the following?
   1. Urination
   2. Salivation
   3. Secretion of mucus
   4. Increased heart rate
      a. 1 and 3
      b. 1, 2, and 3
      c. 2, 3, and 4
      d. 1, 2, 3, and 4

6. A parasympathomimetic agent that intensifies the level of bronchial tone to the point of bronchial constriction and is used in bronchial provocation testing is:
   a. Atropine
   b. Ipratropium
   c. Methacholine
   d. Tiotropium

7. Besides improving lung function in COPD and controlling symptoms, tiotropium may also be useful for controlling symptoms and deterioration of flow rates with:
   a. Nocturnal asthma
   b. Acute bronchitis
   c. Chronic bronchitis
   d. Exercise-induced asthma

8. Which of the following could be assessed to determine the effectiveness of tiotropium bromide?
   1. Keep a count of the number of exacerbations
   2. Keep a count of the number of unscheduled clinic visits
   3. Keep a count of the amount of sputum expectorated during exacerbations
   4. Keep a count of the number of hospitalizations
      a. 1 and 2 only
      b. 2 and 3 only
      c. 1, 2, and 4
      d. 1, 2, 3, and 4

9. In a large, controlled study, patients with COPD who were given a combination of albuterol and ipratropium showed a greater increase in _____ compared with patients given either agent alone.
   a. Slow vital capacity
   b. Vital capacity
   c. Forced expiratory volume at 1 second (FEV_1)
   d. Peak flow rate

10. Combined _____ and _____ therapy may give additive bronchodilating results in COPD and in severe, acute asthma.
    1. Cholinergic
    2. Sympathetic
    3. Anticholinergic
    4. β-Agonist
       a. 1 and 2
       b. 3 and 4
       c. 1, 2 and 4
       d. 2, 3 and 4

11. Which of the following describes quaternary ammonium compounds?
    a. They cross the blood-brain barrier.
    b. They are easily absorbed.
    c. They do not cause CNS changes.
    d. They are distributed throughout the body.

12. Combivent is a combination of which two medications?
    a. Metaproterenol and atropine
    b. Albuterol and atropine
    c. Metaproterenol and ipratropium
    d. Albuterol and ipratropium

13. Which of the following is *true* concerning the sequence of administration of an MDI $β_2$ agonist and an anticholinergic?
    a. $β_2$ agonist is given 30 minutes before an anticholinergic.
    b. $β_2$ agonist is given 45 minutes before an anticholinergic.
    c. The order of administration is not important.
    d. Anticholinergic agent is given before a $β_2$ agonist.

14. Anoro Ellipta is a combination of which two medications?
    a. Albuterol and umeclidinium
    b. Vilanterol and umeclidinium
    c. Vilanterol and ipratropium
    d. Albuterol and tiotropium

15. If ipratropium is delivered as an aerosol nebulizer treatment with a mask, what precautions should be taken?
    a. Pinch the nose of the patient.
    b. Stand outside the room.
    c. Caution the patient not to swallow.
    d. Protect the patient's eyes.

16. Which of the following is a long-acting bronchodilator that can last as long as 32 hours but usually is limited to 16 to 24 hours because of circadian rhythm?
    a. Albuterol
    b. Atropine
    c. Atrovent
    d. Spiriva

17. Which of the following are the only approved anticholinergic agents for inhalation as an aerosol at this time?
    1. Atrovent
    2. Incruse Ellipta
    3. Spiriva
    4. Atropine
        a. 1 and 4
        b. 1 and 3
        c. 2, 3, and 4
        d. 1, 2, and 3

18. The anticholinergic agents ipratropium and tiotropium are indicated for the treatment of which of the following in COPD?
    a. Airflow obstruction
    b. Excess secretions
    c. Air trapping
    d. Nasal congestion

19. The most common side effects seen with aerosolized ipratropium are:
    1. Nasal congestion
    2. Dry mouth
    3. Cough
    4. Excessive salivation
        a. 2 and 3
        b. 1, 2, and 3
        c. 1, 2, and 4
        d. 1, 2, 3, and 4

20. Which three agents are used as triple therapy to help reduce the progression of COPD and improve lung function?
    1. Tiotropium
    2. Salmeterol
    3. Albuterol
    4. Inhaled corticosteroids
        a. 1, 2, and 3
        b. 1, 2, and 4
        c. 2, 3, and 4
        d. 1, 3, and 4

CASE STUDY 1

Jane has a 100 pack-year smoking history. She suffers from a combination of emphysema and chronic bronchitis. Lately, she has been more short of breath than usual, and her dyspnea is accompanied by some expiratory wheezing.

1. What do you think she will respond to better: sympathomimetic bronchodilators or anticholinergic bronchodilators?

2. If you choose combination therapy, such as ipratropium and albuterol, is it better to give each drug separately or as combined therapy?

CASE STUDY 2

A 74-year-old man with a history of COPD has been admitted to the hospital. The patient has been ordered to receive ipratropium.

1. Besides explaining to the patient why he has been prescribed this medication treatment, what would be important to tell the patient concerning a hazard of this drug?

2. The patient asks what would be the best way to administer the drug. What do you tell him?

After trying this technique, the patient requests that he would rather use an SVN because of his familiarity with this method.

3. How should the equipment be set up to avoid drug exposure to the eye?

The patient feels that the mouthpiece will be uncomfortable and requests the use of a mask.

4. What precautions should be taken by the patient to avoid eye contact with the drug?

Several days later, the patient is being discharged from the hospital. The patient has an order to continue ipratropium at home.

5. What aerosol inhalation technique would be best for this patient?

8 Xanthines

CHAPTER OUTLINE

Clinical Indications for Use of Xanthines
Specific Xanthine Agents
General Pharmacologic Properties
Titrating Theophylline Doses
Dosage Schedules
Theophylline Toxicity and Side Effects
Factors Affecting Theophylline Activity
Clinical Application
National Board of Respiratory Care (NBRC) Testing Questions
Case Studies 1 and 2

CHAPTER OBJECTIVES

After answering the following questions, the reader should be able to:

1. Define *xanthine*
2. List all available xanthines used in respiratory therapy
3. Differentiate among the clinical indications of xanthines
4. Differentiate among the uses of xanthines
5. Discuss the proposed theories of activity for xanthines
6. Discuss adverse effects and toxicity of xanthines
7. Be able to clinically assess xanthine therapy

CLINICAL INDICATIONS FOR USE OF XANTHINES

Complete the following questions by writing the answer in the space provided, or by providing a brief answer.

1. List three indications for the use of xanthines.

   a. _____

   b. _____

   c. _____

2. Using the Global Initiative for Chronic Obstructive Lung Disease (GOLD) guidelines, explain when theophylline could be used as a treatment of chronic obstructive pulmonary disease (COPD). Are there any potential problems with its administration?

3. Explain the use of caffeine citrate in premature infants.

4. What benefit does caffeine citrate have over theophylline when treating premature infants for apnea of prematurity?

5. In what two situations would the use of theophylline not be recommended?

   a. _____

   b. _____

SPECIFIC XANTHINE AGENTS

Complete the following questions by writing the correct term in the space provided.

6. List four types of xanthine derivatives used as bronchodilators in obstructive airway diseases. Include both generic and brand names.

   a. _____

   b. _____

   c. _____

   d. _____

7. List three available formulations of theophylline.

   a. _____

   b. _____

   c. _____

GENERAL PHARMACOLOGIC PROPERTIES

8. What are the two proposed mechanisms of action by which theophylline and xanthines reverse airway obstruction?

   a. _____

   b. _____

TITRATING THEOPHYLLINE DOSES

9. Given the following levels of serum theophylline, indicate the effect each level could have on the body.

Micrograms (mg)/Milliliter (mL)	Effect
a. <5	
b. 10-20	
c. >20	
d. >30	
e. 40-45	

10. A range of _____ to _____ μg/mL is now recommended for the treatment of asthma, and a range of _____ to _____ μg/mL is recommended for the treatment of COPD.

11. List six central nervous system (CNS) adverse reactions seen with theophylline treatment.

    a. _____
    b. _____
    c. _____
    d. _____
    e. _____
    f. _____

12. It is important to monitor therapeutic levels of theophylline, because levels higher than 45 μg/mL can cause _____.

DOSAGE SCHEDULES

13. After administering an immediate-release form of theophylline, serum blood levels should be obtained _____ to _____ hours later.

14. After administering a sustained-release form of theophylline, serum blood levels should be measured _____ to _____ hours after the morning dose.

THEOPHYLLINE TOXICITY AND SIDE EFFECTS

15. Match the adverse reactions seen with theophylline with the organ system.

    1. _____ Diuresis
    2. _____ Tachypnea
    3. _____ Nausea
    4. _____ Anxiety
    5. _____ Palpitations
    6. _____ Vomiting
    7. _____ Headache

    a. CNS
    b. Gastrointestinal
    c. Respiratory
    d. Cardiovascular
    e. Renal

16. What precautions should you take when administering theophylline to patients with bronchiectasis or cystic fibrosis?

FACTORS AFFECTING THEOPHYLLINE ACTIVITY

17. *Circle the correct response:* Theophylline is metabolized by the (liver/kidney) and excreted by the (liver/kidney).

CLINICAL APPLICATION

Identify each of the following statements as either true or false.

18. True or False: Theophylline can be used for maintenance therapy in COPD if anticholinergics (ipratropium bromide) and β agonists cannot control the disease.

19. True or False: Most recent guidelines for the pharmacologic management of asthma and COPD suggest theophylline is not indicated as first-line therapy.

20. True or False: Long-acting β_2 agonists, such as salmeterol, give more consistent improvement in lung function on a 12-hour basis in patients with COPD.

21. True or False: A nonbronchodilating effect of theophylline is its ability to strengthen the diaphragm directly.

22. True or False: Theophylline decreases cardiac output and increases pulmonary vascular resistance, thus potentially imposing a greater workload on the heart.

23. True or False: When treating apnea of prematurity, it is better to use theophylline than caffeine, because theophylline is a more potent stimulator of the respiratory system.

24. For use in apnea of prematurity, the recommended loading dose is _____, which is equivalent to 10 mg/mL of caffeine.

25. List three nonbronchodilating effects of theophylline.
    a. _____
    b. _____
    c. _____

NATIONAL BOARD OF RESPIRATORY CARE (NBRC) TESTING QUESTIONS

1. Theophylline is chemically referred to as one of which of the following drugs?
    a. β Blockers
    b. Anticholinergics
    c. Xanthines
    d. Aminophylline agonists

2. Which of the following physiologic effects are found in xanthines?
   1. Improvement in diaphragm muscle endurance
   2. Cardiac stimulation
   3. Diaphragm strengthening
   4. Diuresis
      a. 1 and 3 only
      b. 2 and 4 only
      c. 1, 3, and 4 only
      d. 1, 2, 3, and 4

3. Compared with the β agonists, theophylline has what degree of bronchodilating *effect*?
   a. Weaker
   b. Comparable
   c. Stronger
   d. Much stronger

4. Which of the following make it difficult to titrate theophylline doses?
   1. Theophylline has a narrow therapeutic margin.
   2. Individuals metabolize theophylline at different rates.
   3. Different forms of theophylline are not always equivalent.
   4. The therapeutic effect varies widely among patients.
      a. 1, 2, and 3 only
      b. 2 and 3 only
      c. 2 and 4 only
      d. 1, 2, 3, and 4

5. In the management of asthma, the therapeutic range for serum theophylline is which of the following?
   a. 2 to 12 µg/mL
   b. 5 to 15 µg/mL
   c. 20 to 30 µg/mL
   d. More than 30 µg/mL

6. Cardiovascular side effects associated with theophylline use include which of the following?
   1. Hypotension
   2. Ventricular dysrhythmias
   3. Supraventricular tachycardia
   4. Palpitations
      a. 1 and 2
      b. 2 and 3
      c. 1, 3, and 4
      d. 1, 2, 3, and 4

7. Theophylline may be used to treat which of the following?
   1. Pneumonia
   2. Apnea of prematurity
   3. COPD
   4. Asthma
      a. 1 only
      b. 2 and 3 only
      c. 2, 3, and 4 only
      d. 1, 2, 3, and 4

8. Which of the following conditions can decrease the blood levels of theophylline?
   a. Cirrhosis
   b. Cigarette smoking
   c. Congestive heart failure
   d. Renal failure

9. Methylxanthines are considered first-line agents in the treatment of:
   a. Congestive heart failure
   b. Asthma
   c. COPD
   d. Apnea of prematurity

10. In which of the following formulations is theophylline available?
    1. Aerosol
    2. Intravenous
    3. Oral
    4. Rectal suppository
       a. 1 and 2 only
       b. 2 and 3 only
       c. 2, 3, and 4 only
       d. 1, 2, 3, and 4

11. Why is caffeine considered the drug of choice, compared with theophylline, for treatment of apnea of prematurity?
    1. It penetrates more readily into the cerebrospinal fluid.
    2. It is a more potent stimulator of the CNS.
    3. It has a higher therapeutic index.
    4. It has fewer side effects.
       a. 1 and 2 only
       b. 2 and 3 only
       c. 1, 3, and 4 only
       d. 1, 2, 3, and 4

12. The exact mechanism of action of the methylxanthines is:
    a. Inhibition of phosphodiesterase
    b. Antagonism of adenosine
    c. Release of catecholamines
    d. Unknown

13. What does GOLD recommend for a therapeutic serum level of theophylline when treating COPD patients?
    a. 0 to 5 µg/mL
    b. 5 to 10 µg/mL
    c. 10 to 12 µg/mL
    d. 10 to 20 µg/mL

14. A serum blood theophylline level of 25 µg/mL has been determined for an adult patient in the emergency department. Which of the following effects may be seen with this serum level?
    a. No effects
    b. Cardiac arrhythmias
    c. Nausea and vomiting
    d. Seizures

15. Before using theophylline, which of the following drugs would be of greater benefit to preserve lung function in COPD?
    1. Salmeterol
    2. Formoterol
    3. Arformoterol
    4. Caffeine
       a. 1 only
       b. 2 and 4 only
       c. 1, 2, and 3 only
       d. 1, 3, and 4 only

16. A loading dose of _____ mg/kg of caffeine has been found effective in treating apnea of prematurity.
    a. 0.5
    b. 5
    c. 10
    d. 20

17. It is suggested that giving a patient with COPD theophylline has nonbronchodilating effects. These effects would include:
    1. Ventilatory drive stimulation
    2. Reduced bronchial secretions
    3. Enhanced respiratory muscle function
    4. Antiinflammatory effects
       a. 2 and 4 only
       b. 1 and 3 only
       c. 1, 3, and 4 only
       d. 1, 2, 3, and 4

18. Which of the following factors increase the blood serum levels of theophylline?
    1. Alcohol
    2. Calcium channel blockers
    3. Albuterol
    4. Corticosteroids
       a. 1 and 3
       b. 2 and 3
       c. 1, 2, and 4
       d. 1, 2, 3, and 4

19. Theophylline is contraindicated in which of the following?
    a. Glaucoma
    b. Active peptic ulcer
    c. Diabetes
    d. Acute kidney disease

20. Which of the following are drugs derived from xanthines?
    1. Aminophylline
    2. Theophylline
    3. Octriphylline
    4. Dyphylline
       a. 1 and 2 only
       b. 3 and 4 only
       c. 1, 2, and 4 only
       d. 1, 2, 3, and 4

21. Why is theophylline recommended only as an alternative to inhaled bronchodilators in the treatment of COPD?
    a. It produces excessive secretions.
    b. Acute gastritis is produced.
    c. It reduces forced expiratory volume at 1 second (FEV_1) over long-term administration.
    d. It has potential toxicity because of the narrow therapeutic margin.

22. When administering caffeine, which of the following has the greatest intensity of effects?
    a. Cardiac stimulation
    b. Skeletal muscle stimulation
    c. Diuresis
    d. Smooth muscle relaxation

23. On checking the medical chart of a patient with COPD, you observe the patient has received an immediate-release form of theophylline as a loading dose at 1300. What time should you go back to monitor serum theophylline levels on this patient?
    a. 1430
    b. 1700
    c. 1830
    d. 2200

24. A patient receives a sustained-release form of theophylline in the morning. When should a serum theophylline level be obtained?
    a. 5 to 9 hours later
    b. 13 to 15 hours later
    c. 1 to 2 hours later
    d. 24 hours later

25. How is theophylline removed from the body?
    a. Metabolized by the liver
    b. Removed by the kidney
    c. Removed by the gastrointestinal tract
    d. Metabolized by the kidney

CASE STUDY 1

Joe has been recently diagnosed with COPD. He is 57, has worked in the coal mines since he was 17, and suffers from severe dyspnea. Joe's physician prescribed oxygen for home use at 2 L/min, β agonists, and corticosteroids. Joe has not responded as his physician had hoped. (Joe has had no change in his FEV_1.) Joe's physician has decided to initiate sustained-release theophylline and asks you to calculate the appropriate dose for Joe, who weighs 75 kg and is 6 feet tall.

1. What dose should Joe begin with?

The following day, Joe calls his physician and states that he feels no improvement. The doctor suggests to Joe that he will increase Joe's dose, but he will need to check Joe's theophylline level first.

2. When is the best time to do this?

Joe's serum level comes back as 5 μg/mL. Joe still feels no change or improvement since starting the medication.

3. What should be recommended?

4. Are there any other medications that can be added to his daily regimen?

CASE STUDY 2

Baby Ladarius is a 1500-g, 32-week gestational age newborn who has been in neonatal intensive care for 2 days for laboratory workup and monitoring for irregular breathing and desaturation. Over the last 12 hours, baby Ladarius has had increased episodes of apnea for 30 seconds and bradycardia accompanied by cyanosis. Baby Ladarius requires tactile stimulation to resume breathing. On stimulation, he resumes breathing, and his heart rate and saturation normalize. The respiratory therapist suggests that baby Ladarius has apnea of prematurity, and after consultation with the doctor, the doctor agrees.

1. Based on baby Ladarius's symptoms, what would be considered the first-line medication of choice?

2. The nurse suggests that baby Ladarius receive theophylline to treat his apnea. What do you think about this suggestion?

3. The nurse still believes that theophylline would be better for baby Ladarius because of the nurse's experience with this drug. What else could you tell her to convince her of your suggestion?

4. Okay. The nurse is convinced. What would be the appropriate loading dose of this medication?

5. Twenty-four hours later, baby Ladarius is still having episodes of apnea and bradycardia. What recommendation would you suggest?

9 Mucus-Controlling Drug Therapy

CHAPTER OUTLINE

Key Terms and Definitions
Drug Control of Mucus: A Perspective
Physiology of the Mucociliary System
Nature of Mucus Secretions
Physical Properties of Mucus
Mucoactive Agents
    Mucolytics
    N-Acetyl-L-Cysteine
    Dornase Alfa
    Expectorants
    β Agonists
Mucoregulatory Medications
Antiproteases
Hyperosmolar Saline
Using Mucoactive Therapy with Physical Therapy and Airway Clearance Devices
National Board of Respiratory Care (NBRC) Testing Questions
Case Study

CHAPTER OBJECTIVES

After answering the following questions, the reader should be able to:

1. Define terms that pertain to mucus-controlling drug therapy
2. Interpret the physiology and mechanisms of mucus secretion and clearance
3. Name the types of mucoactive medications and their presumed modes of action
4. Describe the medications approved for the therapy of mucus clearance disorders and their approved indications
5. Identify the contraindications to the use of mucoactive medications
6. Explain the interaction between airway clearance devices or physical therapy and mucoactive medications

KEY TERMS AND DEFINITIONS

Match the following definitions with their terms.

1. _____ Macromolecular description of pseudoplastic material having both viscosity and elasticity

2. _____ Medication that increases cough or ciliary clearance of respiratory secretions

3. _____ The study of deformation and flow of matter in response to an applied stress

4. _____ Medication meant to increase the volume or hydration of airway secretions

a. Elasticity
b. Expectorant
c. Gel
d. Mucin
e. Mucoactive agent
f. Mucokinetic agent
g. Mucolytic agent
h. Mucoregulatory agent
i. Mucospissic
j. Mucus
k. Rheology

5. _____ The principal constituent of mucus

6. _____ Resistance of liquid to sheer forces or energy loss with applied stress

7. _____ Medication that degrades polymers in secretions

8. _____ Secretion, from surface goblet cells and submucosal glands, composed of water, proteins, and glycosylated mucins

9. _____ Term connoting any medication or drug that has an effect on mucus secretion

10. _____ Expectorated secretions that contain respiratory tract, oropharyngeal, and nasopharyngeal secretions, as well as bacteria and products of inflammation, including polymeric DNA and actin

11. _____ A drug that reduces the volume of airway mucus secretion and appears to be especially effective in hypersecretory states

12. _____ Rheologic property characteristic of solids

13. _____ A medication that increases the viscosity of secretions and may be effective in the therapy of bronchorrhea

14. _____ Protein that gives mucus its physical/chemical properties, such as viscoelasticity

15. _____ Referred to as the periciliary layer

16. _____ Sugar that is the individual carbohydrate unit of glycoprotein

17. _____ Purulent material in the airways

l. Sputum
m. Viscosity
n. Glycoprotein
o. Sol
p. Oligosaccharide
q. Phlegm

DRUG CONTROL OF MUCUS: A PERSPECTIVE

18. When should mucoactive therapy be considered?

19. List five factors of mucus that are beneficial regardless of its location.

    a. _____

    b. _____

    c. _____

    d. _____

    e. _____

20. For the mucoactive agents listed, provide the following information:

Drug	Brand Name	Use	Adult Dose
N-acetylcysteine-L-cysteine (NAC)			
Dornase alfa			
Water, saline (0.9%)			
Hyperosmolar saline (3% and 7%)			

PHYSIOLOGY OF THE MUCOCILIARY SYSTEM

21. What are the two airway mucus layers called? Briefly describe each.

    a. _____

    b. _____

22. Explain the difference between mucus and sputum.

23. Complete the following table concerning the effects of various drug groups on mucociliary clearance.

Drug Group	Ciliary Beat	Mucus Production
β-Adrenergic agents		
Cholinergic agents		
Methylxanthines		
Corticosteroids		
Anticholinergics		

NATURE OF MUCUS SECRETIONS

24. List seven factors that can slow mucociliary transport.

    a. _____

    b. _____

    c. _____

    d. _____

    e. _____

    f. _____

    g. _____

25. _____ _____ is considered the most important predisposing factor to airway irritation and mucus hypersecretion, but other factors can include viral infections, pollutants, and genetic predisposition in patients with chronic bronchitis.

26. Briefly describe each of the following disease states and give a reason each may require mucus-controlling drug therapy.

    a. Chronic bronchitis:
    b. Asthma:
    c. Bronchorrhea:
    d. Plastic bronchitis:
    e. Cystic fibrosis (CF):

27. The secretions in CF have very little _____ and are almost entirely composed of _____ _____ derived from neutrophil degradation.

PHYSICAL PROPERTIES OF MUCUS

28. Why is it so difficult for a person with purulent sputum to cough it up?

MUCOACTIVE AGENTS

Mucolytics

29. Discuss two therapeutic options, besides using mucoactive agents, for controlling mucus hypersecretion.

   a. _____

   b. _____

***N*-Acetyl-L-Cysteine**

30. NAC works by disrupting _____ _____ and is more effective in alkaline pH environments (7.0 to 9.0).

31. When administering NAC by aerosol, bronchospasm may occur. The incidence of bronchospasm can be reduced by pretreatment with a _____-_____ bronchodilator.

32. List a nonrespiratory indication for the use of NAC.

Dornase Alfa

33. Why should dornase alfa not be prescribed for patients with bronchiectasis and chronic obstructive pulmonary disease (COPD)?

34. List three indications for the use of dornase alfa:

   a. _____

   b. _____

   c. _____

35. What nebulizers and compressors have been approved for delivery of dornase alfa?

36. What are the brand name, dose, and nebulizer administration requirements for dornase alfa?

37. How would you evaluate the effectiveness of dornase alfa in a patient with CF?

Expectorants

38. Guaifenesin has been approved by the U.S. Food and Drug Administration (FDA) as a bilayer extended-release tablet and as an expectorant called _____ .

β Agonists

39. What disease would benefit from increased expiratory airflow with the use of β agonists?

40. Your patient has been diagnosed with tracheomalacia. She has taken β agonists in the past, but her physician suggested she stop. Can you explain to her why?

MUCOREGULATORY MEDICATIONS

41. The long-term use of a mucoregulatory medication such as ipratropium is associated with a reduction in the volume of mucus secretion in patients with _____ _____ .

ANTIPROTEASES

42. In what disease would antiproteases be helpful in restoring the bacteria-killing capacity of neutrophils?

HYPEROSMOLAR SALINE

43. Why is hyperosmolar saline (hypertonic saline) thought to improve mucociliary transport?

44. A patient with CF has been prescribed hyperosmolar therapy using a 7% hypertonic saline solution administered twice daily (bid). What recommended delivery device should be used for this therapy?

USING MUCOACTIVE THERAPY WITH PHYSICAL THERAPY AND AIRWAY CLEARANCE DEVICES

45. What is the difference between a directed cough and a huff cough?

Identify each of the following statements as either true or false.

46. True or False: Conventional chest physical therapy (CPT) incorporating postural drainage results in significantly greater expectoration than no treatment in patients with CF.

47. True or False: The insufflation-exsufflation device inflates the lungs with positive pressure followed by a negative pressure to simulate a cough.

48. True or False: The active cycle of breathing techniques uses relaxed diaphragmatic breathing and the insufflation-exsufflation device.

49. True or False: Autogenic drainage incorporates staged breathing, starting with small tidal breaths from expiratory reserve volume (ERV), repeated until secretions "collect" in the central airways. It is recommended for patients more than 8 years of age.

50. True or False: Exercise, if tolerated, should be substituted for other bronchial hygiene regimens.

51. With what airway clearance device does the patient breathe through a mouthpiece that delivers high-flow minibursts at rates exceeding 200 cycles/min?

52. Which airway clearance device provides pressure pulses that fill a vest and vibrate the chest wall at variable frequencies applied during the entire respiratory cycle?

53. *Match the descriptions to the appropriate airway clearance method.*

   1. _____ Mr. Cilia is a 69-year-old patient with COPD. He uses this positive airway pressure (PAP) technique as an effective alternative to CPT in expanding the lungs and mobilizing secretions.

   2. _____ Randolph is a 32-year-old patient with CF and uses this device when he is traveling. This device combines positive expiratory pressure (PEP) with high-frequency oscillations at the airway opening.

   3. _____ Robin is a 29-year-old who has CF. She is a salesperson for a pharmaceutical company, travels extensively, and is very motivated. The airway clearance technique she uses incorporates staged breathing starting with small tidal breaths from ERV, repeated until secretions "collect" in the central airways. It is recommended for patients more than 8 years of age.

   4. _____ Ronald is an 18-year-old student with CF, and he is attending his first year of college away from home. Because he is independent and must perform his own therapy, the airway clearance device he uses provides pressure pulses that fill a vest and vibrate the chest wall at variable frequencies applied during the entire respiratory cycle. He uses it for 20-30 minutes per treatment and takes his nebulized medication at the same time.

   5. _____ Alfred is a 22-year-old man with CF. He does not tolerate or like any other device except this one, which provides breaths through a mouthpiece and delivers high-flow minibursts at rates exceeding 200 cycles/min.

   6. _____ Mary is a 44-year-old woman with cerebral palsy. She has poor coughing and limited expiratory airflow. When in the hospital she uses this device, which can generate high-frequency oscillations at the airway opening or on the chest wall.

   7. _____ Lauren is 18 years old and has cerebral palsy and severe scoliosis. This device inflates her lungs with positive pressure, followed by negative pressure to simulate a cough.

   8. _____ Jasmin has just taken a job as a traveling respiratory therapist. Jasmin has CF and believes it would be best to use a technique that allows her not to take equipment with her. Her CF clinic taught her this airway clearance technique. It is a combination of breathing control (relaxed diaphragmatic breathing), thoracic expansion control (deep breaths), and a forced expiration technique from progressively increasing lung volumes.

   a. Chest wall oscillation: The Vest
   b. FLUTTER mucus clearance device
   c. Autogenic drainage
   d. Active cycle of breathing technique
   e. An insufflation-exsufflation device
   f. Pursed-lip breathing
   g. Intrapulmonary percussive ventilation

NATIONAL BOARD OF RESPIRATORY CARE (NBRC) TESTING QUESTIONS

1. A mucokinetic medication is one that:
   a. Increases ciliary clearance of respiratory mucus secretions
   b. Increases the volume or hydration of airway secretions
   c. Degrades polymers in secretions
   d. Increases ciliary activity

2. Pulmozyme is used primarily for:
   a. Chronic bronchitis
   b. Sputum induction
   c. CF
   d. Bronchitis

3. How would you evaluate the effectiveness of dornase alfa in the patient with CF?
   1. Reduction in intravenous (IV) antibiotic use
   2. Reduced need for hospitalizations
   3. Stability of lung function
   4. Reduced number and severity of infectious exacerbations
      a. 1 and 2 only
      b. 3 and 4 only
      c. 1, 3, and 4 only
      d. 1, 2, 3, and 4

4. Which of the following cells or glands is most likely responsible for the majority of mucus secretion?
   a. Ciliated epithelial cells
   b. Goblet cells
   c. Clara cells
   d. Submucosal glands

5. Which of the following forces severely reduces the ability to clear secretions by coughing?
   a. Viscosity
   b. Adhesion
   c. Elasticity
   d. Spinnability

6. Which of the following drugs increases ciliary beat?
   1. β Adrenergics
   2. Cholinergics
   3. Methylxanthines
   4. Corticosteroids
      a. 2 and 4 only
      b. 1 and 3 only
      c. 1, 2, and 3 only
      d. 1, 2, 3, and 4

7. Which of the following is considered the most important predisposing factor to airway irritation and mucus hypersecretion with chronic bronchitis?
   a. Viral infections
   b. Tobacco smoke
   c. Pollutants
   d. Genetic predisposition

8. CF is associated with chronic airway infection, most often caused by:
   a. *Pseudomonas aeruginosa*
   b. *Staphylococcus aureus*
   c. *Streptococcus aureus*
   d. *Haemophilus influenzae*

9. Which of the following are therapeutic options for controlling mucus hypersecretion, other than using mucoactive agents?
   1. Remove causative factors, such as pollution, where possible.
   2. Treat infections.
   3. Optimize tracheobronchial clearance, including the use of bronchodilators.
   4. Incorporate bronchial hygiene measures, such as cough and postural drainage.
      a. 1 and 2 only
      b. 2 and 3 only
      c. 1, 3, and 4 only
      d. 1, 2, 3, and 4

10. Which of the following is considered to be a mucoactive agent?
    a. Dornase alfa
    b. Acetylcysteine
    c. Budesonide
    d. Sodium bicarbonate

11. When administering NAC by aerosol, it is important to include pretreatment with which of the following to reduce the incidence of bronchospasm?
    a. Short-acting beta agonist
    b. Corticosteroid
    c. Cholinergic medication
    d. Expectorant

12. Opened vials of NAC should be:
    a. A purple color
    b. Stored in a refrigerator
    c. Stored in a lighted area that is room temperature
    d. Pink in color

13. Which of the following is suggested equipment for nebulization of dornase alfa?
    1. Hudson Updraft II
    2. Acorn II
    3. Pari LC Jet Plus
    4. Hamilton Fat Boy II
       a. 1 and 4 only
       b. 2 and 4 only
       c. 1, 2, and 3 only
       d. 1, 2, 3, and 4

14. Common side effects with the use of dornase alfa include:
    1. Voice alteration
    2. Pharyngitis
    3. Thrush
    4. Laryngitis
       a. 1 and 3 only
       b. 2 and 4 only
       c. 1, 2, and 3 only
       d. 1, 2, and 4 only

15. NAC can be used to treat overdose of which of the following?
    a. Cocaine
    b. Tylenol
    c. Motrin
    d. Sinutab

16. A patient with CF has been prescribed hyperosmolar therapy using a 7% hypertonic saline solution administered bid. What recommended delivery device should be used for this therapy?
    a. Hudson Updraft II
    b. Ultrasonic Nebulizer
    c. Pari LC Jet Plus
    d. Hamilton Fat Boy II

17. What percent hypertonic saline is recommended for use to induce a cough and improve mucociliary transport and lung function in CF?
    a. 7
    b. 5
    c. 3
    d. 0.9

18. Which of the following assessments is best for drug therapy for respiratory secretions to determine changes in the lung resulting from mucociliary clearance?
    a. FEV_1
    b. Change in lung function over time
    c. Vital capacity
    d. Peak flow rate

19. The surface of the trachea and bronchi include primarily which of the following type(s) of cells?
    1. Columnar epithelium
    2. Ciliated cells
    3. Goblet cells
    4. Pseudostratified cells
       a. 2 and 3 only
       b. 1 and 4 only
       c. 1, 3, and 4 only
       d. 2, 3, and 4 only

20. Which of the following is a reason that NAC should not be used as a mucoactive medication?
    a. The sulfur ingredient disrupts important mucins.
    b. It increases epithelial mucus and chloride secretion.
    c. It does not improve mucus clearance when given as an aerosol.
    d. It swells the mucus and causes reduced expectoration resulting from small airway blockage.

CASE STUDY

Johnny is a 6-year-old boy recently diagnosed with CF. Dr. Choo has just met with Johnny and his parents. They have come to your office for instruction and answers regarding the respiratory care Johnny will be receiving. Dr. Choo has ordered dornase alfa (Pulmozyme) and The Vest airway clearance system for Johnny. Johnny is to return for a follow-up visit in two weeks.

1. The parents want to know what equipment they will need to deliver the dornase alfa to Johnny and how often he should get it.

2. Because the equipment and medication are new to Johnny and his parents, what should you instruct them to do regarding Johnny's physical assessment so they feel more confident with this new therapy?

3. The parents know a child with CF who is 13 years old and does autogenic drainage and percussion and postural drainage, which do not require equipment. Can Johnny be taught this now and use this instead of The Vest?

4. Are any side effects associated with dornase alfa (Pulmozyme)?

5. Johnny has been using The Vest off and on for the past few months, but his parents forget how much pulse frequency to use. They believe it is somewhere about 5 Hz but are unsure. What should the respiratory therapist tell his parents?

6. What if Johnny doesn't tolerate or like The Vest? Can he switch to something else?

10 Surfactant Agents

CHAPTER OUTLINE

Key Terms and Definitions
Identification of Surfactant Preparations
Exogenous Surfactants
    Composition of Pulmonary Surfactant
    Types of Exogenous Surfactant Preparations
Specific Exogenous Surfactant Preparations
    National Board of Respiratory Care (NBRC) Testing Questions
    Case Studies 1 and 2

CHAPTER OBJECTIVES

After answering the following questions, the reader should be able to:

1. Define key terms that pertain to surfactant agents
2. List all available exogenous surfactant agents used in respiratory therapy
3. Describe the mode of action for exogenous surfactant agents
4. Discuss the route of administration for exogenous surfactant agents
5. Recognize hazards and complications of exogenous surfactant therapy
6. Assess the use of surfactant therapy

KEY TERMS AND DEFINITIONS

Complete the following questions by writing the answer in the space provided.

1. A surface-active agent designed to lower surface tension is called a(n) _____.

2. The force caused by the attraction between like molecules, which occur at the liquid-gas interface, and that holds the liquid surface intact, is called _____ _____.

3. Explain why liquid molecules "draw in" on themselves and result in a spherical shape.

4. Laplace's Law describes and quantifies the relationship among:

    a. _____

    b. _____

    c. _____

5. Why is Laplace's Law different in the alveoli?

6. As Laplace's Law applies to the lung, the _____ the surface tension, the greater the compressing force inside the alveolus, which can lead to _____ of the alveolus.

IDENTIFICATION OF SURFACTANT PREPARATIONS

7. Fill in the following table of exogenous surfactant preparations currently approved in the United States.

Drug	Brand Name	Amount in Vial	Initial Dose
Beractant			
Calfactant			
Poractant alfa			
Lucinactant			

EXOGENOUS SURFACTANTS

8. _____ *surfactant* refers to drugs that are preparations formed outside the patient's own body. The key to their use is the _____ _____ of surfactant production.

9. Exogenous surfactant is clinically indicated for the treatment and prevention of _____ in the newborn infant.

10. _____ treatment helps prevent respiratory distress syndrome (RDS) in very-low-birth-weight infants, and in higher-birth-weight infants who have evidence of immature lungs and who are at risk for developing RDS.

11. Retroactive or _____ treatment is for infants who have developed RDS.

Composition of Pulmonary Surfactant
Complete the following questions by writing the answer in the space provided.

12. What is the primary function of surfactant in the lung?

13. Dipalmitoylphosphatidylcholine (DPPC), or _____, is primarily responsible for reduction of alveolar surface tension.

14. What is the major stimulus for surfactant secretion?

15. What is the estimated half-life of surfactant?

16. Surfactant lipids are synthesized and stored in type II alveolar cells in vesicles termed _____ _____.

17. Based on the figure below, what change has occurred to the pressure-volume curve after administration of surfactant to the lung?

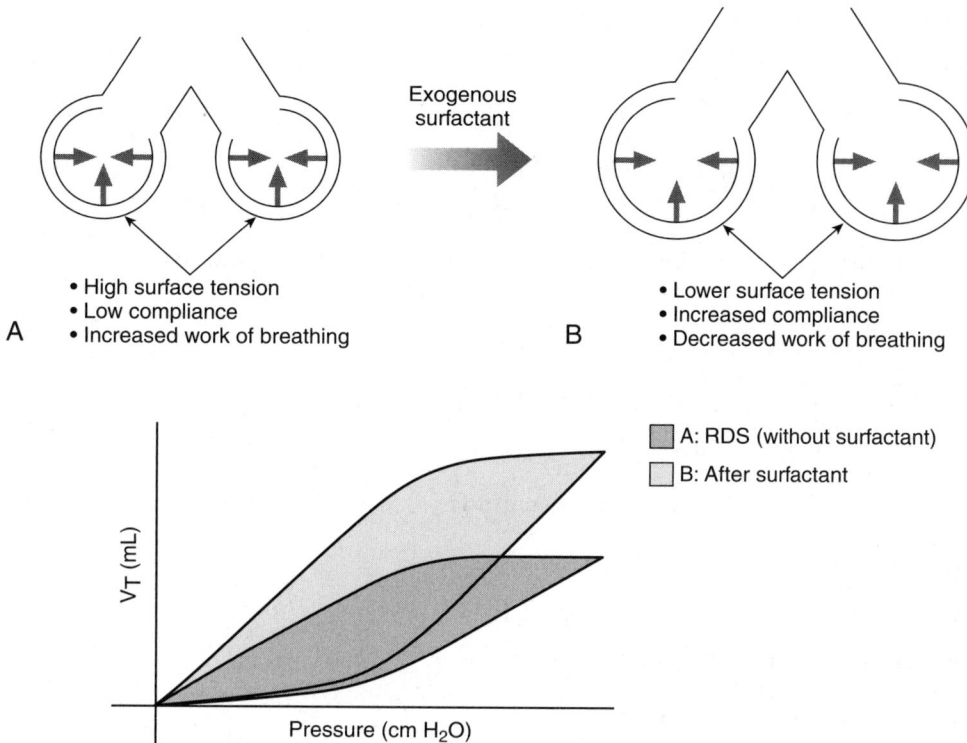

Types of Exogenous Surfactant Preparations
Complete the following questions by writing the answer in the space provided.

18. _____ surfactants are obtained from animals or humans by alveolar wash or from amniotic fluid.

19. Survanta and Infasurf come from _____ lungs, and Curosurf comes from _____ lungs.

SPECIFIC EXOGENOUS SURFACTANT PREPARATIONS

Complete the following questions by writing the answer in the space provided.

20. List two indications for the use of beractant (Survanta)
    a. _____
    b. _____

21. True or False: If a suspension of Survanta has settled, shake the vial for 30 seconds before administration.

22. True or False: Survanta must be refrigerated, but warmed for 20 minutes before administration.

23. True or False: A dose of Survanta is administered through a 5-French catheter placed within the endotracheal tube (ETT).

24. What is the recommended dose of Survanta?

25. List two indications for the use for calfactant (Infasurf).

   a. _____

   b. _____

26. True or False: Repeat doses of Infasurf, up to a total of three doses, can be given 12 hours apart.

27. True or False: Repeat doses of Infasurf as early as 6 hours after the previous dose can be given if the infant is still intubated and requires 30% or greater oxygen for a partial pressure of arterial oxygen (PaO_2) of 80 mm Hg or less.

28. What is the difference in patient positioning between side-port administration and catheter administration of Infasurf?

   a. Side-port administration: _____

   b. Catheter administration: _____

29. What is the recommended dose of Infasurf?

30. List two indications for the use of poractant alfa (Curosurf).

   a. _____

   b. _____

31. Describe how an infant is positioned during administration of Curosurf.

32. What is the recommended dose of Curosurf?

33. List the indication for the use of lucinactant (Surfaxin).

34. Describe in detail how lucinactant is administered.

35. List three observations that would indicate that a newborn infant has responded well to administration of exogenous surfactant:

   a. _____

   b. _____

   c. _____

36. What human recombinant surfactant is being studied for use in acute RDS (ARDS) and can be administered using a mesh nebulizer? _____

NATIONAL BOARD OF RESPIRATORY CARE (NBRC) TESTING QUESTIONS

1. Surfactant accomplishes which of the following?
   a. Decreases lung compliance
   b. Lowers surface tension
   c. Forces pulmonary blood flow to perfuse nonventilated alveoli
   d. Improves mucociliary escalator

2. Which of the following happens as the surface tension of the liquid lining of the alveolus increases?
   a. More pulmonary blood flow perfuses the alveoli.
   b. It becomes more difficult for the alveolus to inflate.
   c. Airway resistance decreases.
   d. More type I cells are produced.

3. Which of the following cells is responsible for surfactant production?
   a. Type I
   b. Type II
   c. Type III
   d. Macrophage

4. Which term describes surfactant preparations from outside the patient's own body?
   a. Endogenous
   b. Exogenous
   c. Synthetic-type
   d. Detergent-type

5. Surfactant is composed of which of the following?
   a. Various amino acids
   b. 10% lipids and 90% proteins
   c. 50% lipids and 50% proteins
   d. 90% lipids and 10% proteins

6. How is exogenous surfactant administered?
   a. Aerosol route
   b. Direct instillation into the trachea
   c. Intravenously (IV)
   d. Parenteral route

7. Which of the following is Laplace's Law as it relates to the alveoli?
   a. 4 × surface tension/radius
   b. 4 × radius/surface tension
   c. 2 × radius/surface tension
   d. 2 × surface tension/radius

8. What would be the initial dose of Infasurf administered for prophylactic treatment of a newborn infant weighing 1 kg?
   a. 2.5 mL in four equally divided doses
   b. 3.0 mL in two equally divided doses
   c. 3.5 mL in four equally divided doses
   d. 4.0 mL in two equally divided doses

9. What is the reason that exogenously administered surfactant is successful in replacing surfactant in the lung after one or two doses?
   a. It is taken into the surfactant pool and recycled.
   b. Blood flow improves and allows more surfactant to be produced.
   c. It completely covers the inside of the alveoli surface.
   d. It improves compliance and increases oxygenation, and thus produces more surfactant.

10. Which of the following is primarily responsible for reduction of alveolar surface tension?
    a. Sphingomyelin
    b. Surfactant protein D
    c. Lecithin
    d. Surfactant protein A

11. The major stimulus for surfactant secretion is believed to be:
    a. Baroreceptors
    b. Chemoreceptors
    c. Pulmonary artery blood flow
    d. Lung inflation

12. What is the recommended dose for Surfaxin?
    a. 2 mL/kg birth weight
    b. 3 mL/kg birth weight
    c. 4.8 mL/kg birth weight
    d. 5.8 mL/kg birth weight

13. Prophylactic Infasurf treatment is indicated for:
    a. Term infants with meconium aspiration syndrome (MAS)
    b. Infants less than 29 weeks of gestational age at risk for developing RDS
    c. Infants with group B streptococcus pneumonia (GBS)
    d. Infants more than 72 hours of age at risk for developing RDS

14. A respiratory therapist is about to administer Infasurf by intratracheal catheter. Appropriate positioning of the infant includes:
    a. Prone position for all doses, first with head down 30 degrees, then head up 30 degrees
    b. Right and left side dependent after each dose, first with head down 30 degrees, then head up 30 degrees
    c. Supine position for all doses first with head down 30 degrees, then head up 30 degrees
    d. Different positioning after each dose: prone, supine, right and left dependent

15. Which of the following procedures should occur immediately after administration of Survanta through a 5-French catheter?
    a. The patient should be turned to the opposite side and the second dose administered.
    b. On removal of the catheter, the infant should be manually ventilated for 30 seconds.
    c. On removal of the catheter, the infant should be manually ventilated for 2 to 5 minutes.
    d. On removal of the catheter, the infant should be placed back on mechanical ventilation in the prone position.

16. Two hours after administration of exogenous surfactant, an infant receiving mechanical ventilation shows an increase in exhaled tidal volume, from 4 to 8 mL/kg of body weight, with no change in pressure delivery. These findings would indicate:
    a. Reduced airway resistance
    b. Increased lung compliance
    c. Increased work of breathing
    d. The need to administer another dose of surfactant

17. An intubated infant just received a dose of Curosurf through a 5-French catheter. The infant is being hand ventilated with 90% oxygen. Suddenly, the infant's heart rate drops from 140 to 75 beats/min, Spo_2 (oxygen saturation as determined by pulse oximetry) decreases from 89% to 70%, and work of breathing and retractions increase. The respiratory therapist should make which of the following recommendations:
    a. Extubate and manually ventilate the infant.
    b. Turn the infant so the opposite lung is dependent.
    c. Suction the ETT.
    d. Reconnect the infant to the ventilator.

18. The respiratory therapist reports to the physician that an infant has had a good response to administration of Curosurf, as indicated by:
    1. Increase in Pao₂
    2. Increase in Paco₂
    3. Increase in lung compliance
        a. 1 only
        b. 2 and 3 only
        c. 1 and 3 only
        d. 1, 2, and 3

19. Natural surfactant is obtained from:
    1. Lungs of cows
    2. Lungs of pigs
    3. Lungs of horses
        a. 1 only
        b. 1 and 2 only
        c. 2 and 3 only
        d. 1, 2, and 3

20. Survanta administered as a rescue treatment for infants with evidence of RDS should occur:
    a. Within 8 hours of birth
    b. Immediately after birth
    c. Within 2 hours of birth
    d. Within 1 hour of birth

21. How much Survanta should be administered for prophylactic treatment of a newborn weighing 700 g?
    a. 2.8 mL
    b. 2.1 mL
    c. 4.0 mL
    d. 4.2 mL

22. A mechanically ventilated newborn infant is receiving Curosurf through an ETT. The respiratory therapist observes that the ETT has become obstructed during instillation, and the infant has desaturated and become bradycardic. Which of the following is recommended?
    a. Increase positive end expiratory pressure (PEEP)
    b. Increase fraction of inspired oxygen (Fio₂)
    c. Increase inspiratory time
    d. Manually ventilate

23. Which of the following is a new synthetic surfactant currently being studied for the treatment of ARDS?
    a. Pulmosurf
    b. Alveolarsurf
    c. Surfnturf
    d. Aerosurf

24. A respiratory therapist has given one dose of exogenous surfactant in the position of right lateral recumbent. The catheter has been removed from the ETT, and the infant is now being manually ventilated with 100% oxygen for 1 minute. After this, a second dose will be given using the same protocol but in the position of left lateral recumbent. This would indicate which of the following exogenous surfactants was most likely given?
    a. Curosurf
    b. Exosurf
    c. Survanta
    d. Infasurf

25. After administration of Infasurf, which of the following clinical changes would indicate improvement in lung mechanics?
    1. Increased compliance
    2. Reduced body temperature
    3. Decreased work of breathing
    4. Reduction in pulmonary secretions
        a. 1 and 3 only
        b. 1, 2, and 3 only
        c. 2, 3, and 4 only
        d. 1, 2, and 4 only

CASE STUDY 1

A male newborn infant with a gestational age of 26 weeks and birth weight of 900 g is in the neonatal intensive care unit (NICU). The 4-hour-old infant has been diagnosed with RDS and is intubated, and has been receiving mechanical ventilation since birth. The decision has been made to administer Survanta. This baby fits the protocol's inclusion criteria, and you have been asked to talk to the parents about this decision.

1. How would you explain to the parents why exogenous surfactant is needed?

2. The parents would like to know how you will determine whether their child is getting better after administration of exogenous surfactant. What do you tell them?

After talking with you, the parents consent to the treatment. You return to the NICU and prepare to administer Survanta.

3. You notice that settling has occurred within the vial. How should it be mixed?

4. How much of the 8-mL vial will the infant require for the first dose if you are administering it through a side-port adaptor?

5. How would you position the baby for each dose?

6. You return to the parents and explain the procedure to them. They ask: "What will happen if he doesn't get better? Can he receive more surfactant?" What would you tell them?

CASE STUDY 2

A 25-week gestational age newborn weighing 600 g has been intubated with a 2.5-mm ETT and is receiving mechanical ventilation. Current ventilator settings are peak inspiratory pressure 20 cm H_2O, exhaled tidal volume 4 mL, inspiratory time 3 seconds, respiratory rate 40/min, positive end-expiratory pressure 4 cm H_2O, Fio_2 0.80. Physical assessment includes pulse 142/min, blood pressure 38/24 mm Hg, Spo_2 85%, temperature 99.6° F. A recent chest radiograph shows findings supportive of RDS. Based on the infant's current ventilatory support and chest x-ray finding, it is decided to administer Curosurf.

1. What is the recommended initial dose of Curosurf that should be administered?

2. What is the protocol for administration of Curosurf?

3. The infant has now received two doses of Curosurf. Over this period of time, the pressure-volume (PV) curve has changed from A to B, as imaged in the figure. Curve A represents when the infant was first mechanically ventilated, and curve B represents the PV curve after the second dose of Curosurf. What change in lung mechanics has occurred that is represented in PV curve B?

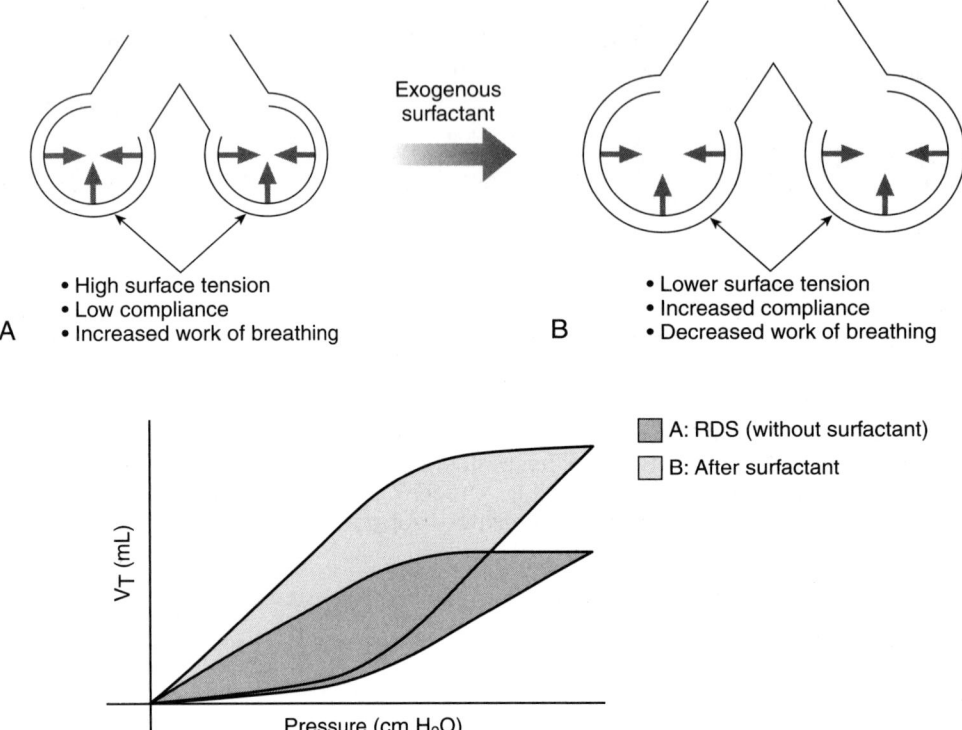

4. Based on the changes seen in curve B in the image in question #3, what are three potential complications that may develop?

   a. _____

   b. _____

   c. _____

11 Corticosteroids in Respiratory Care

CHAPTER OUTLINE

Key Terms and Definitions
Clinical Indication for Use of Inhaled Corticosteroids
Physiology of Corticosteroids
    Identification and Source
Nature of the Inflammatory Response
Inflammation in the Airway
Aerosolized Corticosteroids
Pharmacology of Corticosteroids
Hazards and Side Effects of Steroids
Clinical Application
    Use of Corticosteroids in Chronic Obstructive Pulmonary Disease
National Board of Respiratory Care (NBRC) Testing Questions
Case Studies 1, 2, and 3

CHAPTER OBJECTIVES

After answering the following questions, the reader should be able to:

1. Define key terms that pertain to corticosteroids
2. Discuss the indications for inhaled corticosteroid use
3. List all available inhaled corticosteroids used in respiratory therapy
4. Differentiate among specific corticosteroid formulations
5. Describe the route of administration available for corticosteroids
6. Describe the mode of action for corticosteroids
7. Discuss the effect corticosteroids have on the white blood cell count
8. Discuss the effect corticosteroids have on β receptors
9. Differentiate between systemic and local side effects of corticosteroids
10. Discuss the use of corticosteroids in the treatment of asthma and chronic obstructive disease
11. Be able to assess corticosteroid use in patient care

KEY TERMS AND DEFINITIONS

Complete the following questions by writing the answer in the space provided.

1. The hyperglycemia resulting from steroids' increasing plasma glucose levels through the breakdown of proteins is called _____ _____.

2. Substances produced within the body are called _____.

3. A gamma globulin produced by cells in the respiratory tract is _____.

4. This hormone-type substance, an inflammatory mediator and part of the arachidonic acid cascade, is called _____.

5. Also known as glucocorticoids, _____ produce an antiinflammatory response in the body.

6. Chemicals secreted by the adrenal cortex are called _____ _____ _____.

7. Substances produced outside the body, for administration inside the body, are called _____.

8. Inflammatory process chemicals, produced and released by the body in response to stimuli, are called _____ _____.

CLINICAL INDICATION FOR USE OF INHALED CORTICOSTEROIDS

Complete the following questions by writing the answer in the space provided.

9. List two formulations in which inhaled corticosteroids are available.

    a. _____

    b. _____

10. At what level of care in asthma, as defined by the National Asthma Education and Prevention Program (NAEPP) Expert Panel Report 3 *Guidelines for the Diagnosis and Management of Asthma—Update on Selected Topics*, are corticosteroids clinically indicated?

11. In severe asthma, both inhaled corticosteroids and _____ corticosteroids can be used together.

12. List two clinical indications for intranasal aerosolized corticosteroids.

    a. _____

    b. _____

13. Match the following aerosolized corticosteroids for oral inhalation with their brand name.

    Drug
    1. _____ Mometasone furoate
    2. _____ Beclomethasone dipropionate HFA
    3. _____ Fluticasone propionate/salmeterol
    4. _____ Ciclesonide
    5. _____ Budesonide/formoterol fumarate HFA
    6. _____ Fluticasone propionate
    7. _____ Flunisolide hemihydrate HFA
    8. _____ Budesonide
    9. _____ Mometasone furoate/formoterol fumarate HFA

    Brand Name
    a. AeroSpan
    b. QVAR
    c. Pulmicort Flexhaler, Pulmicort Respules
    d. Asmanex HFA, Asmanex Twisthaler
    e. Advair HFA, Advair Diskus
    f. Symbicort
    g. Flovent HFA, Flovent Diskus
    h. Alvesco
    i. Dulera

14. Match the following aerosolized corticosteroids for intranasal delivery with their brand name.

    Drug
    1. _____ Triamcinolone acetonide
    2. _____ Ciclesonide
    3. _____ Fluticasone
    4. _____ Budesonide
    5. _____ Mometasone furoate
    6. _____ Fluticasone furoate
    7. _____ Beclomethasone

    Brand Name
    a. Nasonex
    b. Beconase AQ
    c. Rhinocort Aqua
    d. Flonase
    e. Nasacort AQ
    f. Veramyst
    g. Omnaris

PHYSIOLOGY OF CORTICOSTEROIDS

Identification and Source

15. Glucocorticoids, often referred to simply as *steroids,* exert an _____ effect in the body.

16. List two side effects of glucocorticoids.

    a. _____

    b. _____

17. What is a primary reason for using aerosolized glucocorticoids versus systemic ones?

18. To withdraw an adrenally suppressed patient from oral corticosteroid treatment, the oral agent is tapered off slowly, while _____ corticosteroids are started.

NATURE OF THE INFLAMMATORY RESPONSE

19. Name two of the most common inflammatory lung diseases.

    a. _____

    b. _____

20. Give a description of each category of the triple response to inflammation.

    a. _____

    b. _____

    c. _____

INFLAMMATION IN THE AIRWAY

21. Evidence indicates that the early asthmatic response is caused by _____-dependent activation of airway mast cells.

22. List four symptoms that, in an acute state, the asthmatic patient will exhibit.

    a. _____

    b. _____

    c. _____

    d. _____

AEROSOLIZED CORTICOSTEROIDS

23. What are the two most common methods used for the delivery of inhaled corticosteroids?

    a. _____

    b. _____

24. Beclomethasone dipropionate (QVAR) has been reformulated with an HFA propellant; it has a lung deposition measured at _____% to _____% of the emitted dose.

25. Flunisolide hemihydrate HFA (Aerospan) is marketed with a built-in _____ device.

26. Flunisolide shows a peak plasma level after inhalation between 2 and 60 minutes, indicating good _____ from the lungs.

27. Flovent is available in what two forms?

    a. _____

    b. _____

28. What is the benefit of using budesonide in the form of Pulmicort Respules compared with the Pulmicort Flexhaler?

29. Because ciclesonide is a prodrug, it has been shown to decrease the development of _____ _____ in the mouth.

30. What two drugs are contained within the dry powder inhaler (DPI) Advair?

    a. _____

    b. _____

31. What two drugs make up Symbicort?

    a. _____

    b. _____

32. Oral inhalation of glucocorticoids is available for the control of _____ and _____. Intranasal administration is for _____.

PHARMACOLOGY OF CORTICOSTEROIDS

33. Steroids suppress the inflammatory response by what three general pathways?

    a. _____

    b. _____

    c. _____

34. Besides suppression of the inflammatory response, what is another benefit of steroids?

HAZARDS AND SIDE EFFECTS OF STEROIDS

35. List six side effects associated with systemic administration of corticosteroids.

   a. _____

   b. _____

   c. _____

   d. _____

   e. _____

   f. _____

36. List three ways to minimize the local side effects of inhaled steroid administration.

   a. _____

   b. _____

   c. _____

CLINICAL APPLICATION

Use of Corticosteroids in Chronic Obstructive Pulmonary Disease

37. What are the different patterns in the inflammatory cells in chronic obstructive pulmonary disease (COPD) and those in asthma?

38. In asthma, to verify peak expiratory flow rate, a _____ _____ _____ should be used.

39. When a patient is using a metered dose inhaler (MDI) for inhaled corticosteroids, the patient should use a _____ _____ to enhance deposition in the lungs.

40. List five respiratory care assessments you would perform before the treatment of an inhaled corticosteroid.

   a. _____

   b. _____

   c. _____

   d. _____

   e. _____

41. List two respiratory care assessments you would perform with long-term treatment of an inhaled corticosteroid.

   a. _____

   b. _____

NATIONAL BOARD OF RESPIRATORY CARE (NBRC) TESTING QUESTIONS

1. Corticosteroids are naturally secreted by which of the following?
   a. Thymal cortex: outer zone
   b. Adrenal cortex: outer zone
   c. Adrenal cortex: inner zone
   d. Thymal cortex: inner zone

2. Which of the following are clinical indicators for intranasal aerosol steroids?
   1. Seasonal allergies
   2. Acute persistent mild asthma
   3. Perennial allergies
   4. Acute exacerbation of COPD
      a. 1 and 3 only
      b. 2 and 4 only
      c. 1, 2, and 3 only
      d. 1, 2, 3, and 4

3. Corticosteroids are described as which of the following?
   a. Bronchodilators
   b. Smooth muscle dilators
   c. Antiinflammatory agents
   d. Lipid-soluble agents

4. Which of the following occurs during an asthma attack?
   1. Bronchospasm
   2. Release of epinephrine
   3. Mucosal edema
   4. Increased secretions
      a. 1, 2, 3, and 4
      b. 1, 2, and 3 only
      c. 1, 3, and 4 only
      d. 2, 3, and 4 only

5. Fluticasone propionate and salmeterol are drugs that are found in:
   a. Azmacort
   b. Advair HFA
   c. Symbicort
   d. QVAR

6. Which of the following are general symptoms of inflammation?
   1. Redness
   2. Swelling
   3. Heat
   4. Pain
      a. 1 and 2
      b. 3 and 4
      c. 2, 3, and 4
      d. 1, 2, 3, and 4

7. Regardless of the type of asthma, allergic or nonallergic, the major effector cells of the inflammatory response are which of the following?
   1. Neutrophil
   2. Mast cell
   3. Macrophage
   4. Eosinophil
      a. 1 and 3
      b. 2 and 4
      c. 1, 3, and 4
      d. 1, 2, and 4

8. Which of the following describes aerosol administration of corticosteroids?
   a. It is associated with no side effects.
   b. It produces severe side effects.
   c. It results in more systemic than local side effects.
   d. It results in minimal side effects

9. Which of the following minimizes local side effects associated with use of inhaled corticosteroids?
   a. Use of a spacer device
   b. Rinsing the mouth after each treatment
   c. Taking the lowest dose possible
   d. All the above

10. Which of the following is recommended to avoid complicating side effects seen with systemic treatment with steroids?
    a. Reduce dosage
    b. Reduce number of days of treatment
    c. Switch to aerosol administration
    d. Switch to every-other-day administration

11. Early asthmatic response is caused by:
    a. Eosinophils
    b. Neutrophils
    c. Plasma leakage
    d. Immunoglobulin E

12. The common side effects of inhaled steroids include:
    1. Oral thrush
    2. Excessive oral secretions
    3. Dysphonia
    4. Yellowing of the teeth
       a. 1 and 4 only
       b. 1 and 3 only
       c. 1, 2, and 3 only
       d. 1, 2, 3, and 4

13. Symbicort is a combination of:
    a. Albuterol and fluticasone
    b. Budesonide and formoterol
    c. Atrovent and fluticasone
    d. Budesonide and salmeterol

14. If a drug such as flunisolide shows a peak plasma level quickly, within 2 minutes, this would indicate:
    a. Reduced removal from the body by the kidney
    b. Excessive dose delivery
    c. Excessive oropharyngeal deposition
    d. Good absorption by the lungs

15. Mometasone and formoterol are drugs found in:
    a. Dulera
    b. Symbicort
    c. Advair
    d. QVAR

16. One of the primary reasons for using aerosolized glucocorticoids is to minimize _____ suppression.
    a. Eosinophil
    b. Neutrophil
    c. Adrenal
    d. White blood cell

17. A patient who has severe asthma has been prescribed corticosteroids for her treatment. She wants to know which type of corticosteroid she should use that will have minimal adverse effects. You would suggest:
    1. Inhaled
    2. Systemic
    3. Pill
    4. Injection
       a. 1
       b. 1 and 2
       c. 1, 3, and 4
       d. 1, 2, and 4

18. What is one advantage of using ciclesonide over other inhalation steroids?
    a. It decreases the development of *Candida albicans* in the mouth.
    b. It has a greater percent deposition in the lung.
    c. It is flavored and therefore reduces irritability in the oral cavity.
    d. It comes with a built-in holding chamber.

19. The best way to monitor changes in peak expiratory flow rate in a person with asthma who is taking inhaled steroids is to:
    a. Measure monthly steroid levels
    b. Keep a journal detailing nocturnal sleeping pattern
    c. Use a peak flow meter
    d. Use 1 month on and 1 month off treatment to identify wheezing patterns

20. To prevent the need to increase inhaled corticosteroid use in a person who is currently receiving low-dose inhaled steroids, which of the following is recommended?
    a. Short-term course of antibiotics
    b. Systemic corticosteroid administration
    c. Short-acting anticholinesterase medication
    d. Long-acting β_2 agonist

CASE STUDY 1
Asthma

Mrs. Peacock has been prescribed beclomethasone dipropionate (QVAR) 40 μg/puff (two puffs two times daily), as treatment for moderate asthma.

1. How much QVAR will she receive in a 24-hour period?

2. Mrs. Peacock has never used an MDI with a spacer device. When you are instructing her in the use of her MDI, what points must you cover?

3. Mrs. Peacock wants to know whether she should increase the number of puffs of QVAR if she begins having shortness of breath and more coughing and wheezing. What do you tell her?

CASE STUDY 2
Asthma

(Information on the NAEPP can be accessed at http://www.nhlbi.nih.gov/guidelines/asthma/index.htm)

Zach is a 29-year-old male with asthma who lives in Atlanta. It is springtime, so the pollen is extremely thick. He monitors himself and is considered at present to require step 1 care in his management of asthma. When he has minor exacerbations, he uses his MDI of albuterol. Over the past 2 weeks, he has had several more exacerbations. His symptoms include nighttime coughing, increased wheezing, and tightness in his chest, and his peak expiratory flow rate has dropped 22%. He has come to the doctor's office, and the asthma educator sees him.

1. What should the educator recommend to Zach?

Zach has agreed to this change. It is now 4 days later and he is not getting better. In fact, his nighttime symptoms are worse, and he is not able to sleep through the night because of severe coughing. Seeking advice, he calls the asthma educator.

2. What is the next recommendation for Zach?

3. Zach has never taken the medication recommended in question 2. What would you tell him about the formulation and dosage?

CASE STUDY 3
Chronic Obstructive Lung Disease

(Information on the Global Initiative for Chronic Obstructive Lung Disease [GOLD] guidelines can be accessed at http://www.goldcopd.com/)

Charles is a 69-year-old patient in the emergency department who has complaints of increasing shortness of breath and increased coughing with increased sputum production. His sputum is more purulent in appearance, and he has a fever. His respiratory rate is 34 breaths/min, and his pulse oximetry oxygen saturation (SpO_2) is 90%. He is taking albuterol by MDI at home. He states that he used his MDI but continues to be short of breath. His past medical history includes that he was a coal miner for 10 years and then became a laborer, cutting wood in a lumber yard. He has been admitted to the hospital several times over the past five years. He further states he used to smoke but gave that up a year ago. After the respiratory therapist and doctor have talked, they agree that the patient has COPD.

1. In this scenario, list four assessments that would indicate the patient may have COPD.

   a. _____

   b. _____

   c. _____

   d. _____

2. A laboratory report from a sample drawn earlier on admission has returned. Based on this patient's history, what would you expect would be a common inflammatory cell in this laboratory report?

3. Charles has been prescribed an inhaled corticosteroid after he is admitted to the hospital. He wants to know whether the corticosteroid will help his pulmonary function. What do you tell him?

4. Charles has been admitted to the hospital and has had a pulmonary function testing. Andy has been diagnosed with stage 2 moderate COPD. What are three characteristics of stage 2 moderate COPD?

   a. _____

   b. _____

   c. _____

5. After several days, Charles is discharged. What respiratory home medications should he use to prevent future exacerbations?

6. Besides the respiratory home medications, what other pharmacologic treatment should be recommended based on his diagnosis and his age?

12 Nonsteroidal Antiasthma Agents

CHAPTER OUTLINE

Key Terms and Definitions
National Board of Respiratory Care (NBRC) Testing Questions
Case Study

CHAPTER OBJECTIVES

After answering the following questions, the reader should be able to:

1. Define terms that pertain to nonsteroidal antiasthmatic agents
2. Discuss the indications for nonsteroidal antiasthma agents
3. List available nonsteroidal antiasthma agents used in respiratory therapy
4. Differentiate among the specific nonsteroidal antiasthma agents
5. Describe the routes of administration available for various nonsteroidal antiasthma agents
6. Describe the mechanism of action for various nonsteroidal antiasthma agents
7. Discuss the use of nonsteroidal antiasthma agents in the treatment of asthma

KEY TERMS AND DEFINITIONS

Complete the following questions by writing the answer in the space provided.

1. Connective tissue cells that contain heparin and histamine are called _____ _____.

2. Cromolyn is a _____ _____ _____ as a prophylactic treatment for asthma.

3. Chemical mediators that cause inflammation are called _____.

4. An agent that blocks the inflammatory response in asthma is called a(n) _____.

5. _____ is a gamma globulin that is produced by cells in the respiratory tract.

6. Alternatives to low-dose corticosteroids in step 2 asthma include _____ and _____.

7. In infants and children, _____ are an alternative to inhaled corticosteroids in step 2 asthma because of their safety profiles.

8. All the nonsteroidal antiasthma drugs described in this chapter are _____, not relievers, and should never be used during an acute exacerbation of asthma.

9. Describe a clinical situation in which the use of a controller medication is indicated.

10. The following is a list of drugs that are either controllers or relievers. *Place a C next to the drug if it is a controller and an R if it is a reliever.*

    a. Inhaled corticosteroids: _____

    b. Oral corticosteroids: _____

    c. Leukotriene modifiers: _____

    d. Cromolyn sodium: _____

    e. Inhaled short-acting adrenergic bronchodilators: _____

11. List three components of asthma.

    a. _____

    b. _____

    c. _____

12. List three modes of action of cromolyn sodium.

    a. _____

    b. _____

    c. _____

13. It may take _____ to _____ weeks of cromolyn sodium use before reducing the concomitant therapy of bronchodilator or steroid use.

14. True or False: Cromolyn sodium has no bronchodilating action and should not be used during acute bronchospasm.

15. Besides its use in asthma, list two other indications for the use of cromolyn.

    a. _____

    b. _____

16. Name three antileukotriene agents that have been approved for use.

    a. _____

    b. _____

    c. _____

17. What is the indication for Zileuton (Zyflo)?

18. Zyflo is approved for children _____ years of age and older.

19. The recommended dosage of Zyflo for asthma is _____.

20. Two drugs that Zyflo interacts with are _____ and _____.

21. Accolate has been approved for children aged _____ years and older.

22. Accolate inhibits asthma reactions induced by _____, cold air, _____, and aspirin.

23. The dose of Accolate for children 5 to 11 years of age is to take an oral _____-mg tablet twice daily; for children 12 years of age and older, an oral _____-mg tablet to take twice daily is available.

24. Instruct the child to take Accolate _____ hour before eating or _____ hours after eating, because food reduces mean bioavailability.

25. Singulair is the one antileukotriene agent that has been approved for children as young as _____ years of age.

26. Singulair is available in _____ and _____ form and can be taken with or without meals.

27. Singular metabolism is accomplished primarily by the _____ and excreted by the _____.

28. In moderate asthma, a combination of _____ and _____ results in greater lung function.

29. List the triggers for which antileukotrienes are particularly useful in controlling asthma.

    a. _____

    b. _____

    c. _____

30. Asthma guidelines agree that _____ are the most effective antiinflammatory drugs for use in asthma, and they have broader antiinflammatory activity than the more limited effect of the antileukotrienes.

31. A link appears to exist between respiratory syncytial virus (RSV) and asthma. The use of _____ blocks these mediators in asthma, as well as in RSV infection.

32. Briefly describe the mechanism of action of omalizumab (Xolair).

33. True or False: Xolair is not a replacement for corticosteroids.

34. True or False: Xolair is a prophylactic agent for uncontrolled moderate to severe persistent asthma.

35. True or False: Asthma rescue agents may need to be increased with the use of Xolair.

36. List seven advantages of antileukotriene drug therapy.

    a. _____

    b. _____

    c. _____

    d. _____

    e. _____

    f. _____

    g. _____

37. List six disadvantages of antileukotriene drug therapy.

    a. _____

    b. _____

    c. _____

    d. _____

    e. _____

    f. _____

NATIONAL BOARD OF RESPIRATORY CARE (NBRC) TESTING QUESTIONS

1. If a patient experiences an asthma attack as a result of exposure to cats, the asthma would be categorized as which of the following?
   a. Intrinsic
   b. Extrinsic
   c. Autoimmune
   d. Intangible

2. Airway obstruction that occurs with asthma is the result of:
   1. Bronchoconstriction
   2. Mucosal swelling
   3. Increased secretion production
   4. Excessive blood flow to the lungs
      a. 1 and 2 only
      b. 2 and 4 only
      c. 1, 2, and 3 only
      d. 1, 2, 3, and 4

3. Release of cytokines during an allergic response does which of the following?
   a. Cytokines release B lymphocytes.
   b. Cytokines cause sloughing and death of eosinophils.
   c. Endothelial adhesion molecules are upregulated.
   d. Pulmonary vascular resistance is increased and leads to vascular congestion.

4. Which of the following is a mast cell stabilizer?
   1. Cromolyn sodium
   2. Montelukast
   3. Zatirlukast
   4. Omalizumab
      a. 1 only
      b. 2 and 4 only
      c. 1, 2, and 3 only
      d. 1, 2, 3, and 4

5. Cromolyn sodium is used to prevent which of the following?
   a. Inflammatory response
   b. Excessive accumulation of eosinophils
   c. Intrinsic asthma
   d. Reduction of nitric oxide response to asthma

6. The mechanism of action for Accolate is considered to be which of the following?
   a. 5-Lipoxygenase (5-LO) inhibitor
   b. Mast cell stabilizer
   c. Leukotriene receptor antagonist
   d. Leukotriene receptor agonist

7. Cromolyn can be used for the treatment of which of the following?
   a. Exacerbation of chronic obstructive pulmonary disease (COPD)
   b. Seasonal rhinitis
   c. Angiotensin-converting enzyme inhibitor (ACEI)-induced cough
   d. Flu-like symptoms within 2 days of onset

8. The ampoule or vial of cromolyn sodium contains 20 mg or 2 mL of aqueous solution, which is what percent solution?
   a. 1
   b. 2
   c. 3
   d. 4

9. You have determined extubation is not possible, owing to glottis swelling. The physician asks for your suggestion regarding medication choices, which will be given now to aid in the extubation process, which will happen tomorrow. What would you suggest?
   a. Metered dose inhaler (MDI) corticosteroids via endotracheal tube (ETT)
   b. Corticosteroids via oral gastric tube
   c. Intravenous corticosteroids
   d. MDI albuterol

10. Omalizumab (Xolair) can be given to children:
    a. 0 to 4 years of age
    b. 5 to 11 years of age
    c. 12 years of age or older
    d. Any age with approval from treating physician

11. For cromolyn sodium, it may take _____ to _____ weeks for improvement in patients' symptoms, allowing a decrease in concomitant therapy, such as bronchodilator or steroid use.
    a. 1 to 3
    b. 2 to 4
    c. 4 to 6
    d. 8 to 9

12. The antileukotriene modifier that is approved for children younger than 5 years of age is:
    a. Zyflo
    b. Singulair
    c. Accolate
    d. Xolair

13. Which of the following should be monitored once per month when taking Zyflo?
    a. Nitric oxide
    b. Liver enzymes
    c. Kidney enzymes
    d. Pulmonary function tests

14. Drugs that interact with Zyflo and may require dosing adjustment of Zyflo include:
    1. Theophylline
    2. Beclomethasone
    3. Cromolyn sodium
    4. Warfarin
       a. 1 and 4 only
       b. 2 and 3 only
       c. 1 and 2 only
       d. 2 and 4 only

15. For treatment of chronic asthma, a combination of _____ and _____ results in greater lung function than when these drugs are taken separately.
    a. β_2 Agonist and steroid
    b. β_2 Agonist and cromolyn sodium
    c. Corticosteroid and antileukotriene
    d. β_2 Agonist and antileukotriene

16. Concerning exercise-induced asthma, which of the following promotes the generation of leukotrienes that result in bronchoconstriction?
    a. Cooling and drying of the airway
    b. Increased blood flow to the lungs
    c. Airflow increase irritating goblet cells
    d. Increased body temperature producing excessive mucus production

17. Antileukotrienes are particularly useful in controlling asthma resulting from certain triggers, including which of the following?
    1. Exercise-induced asthma
    2. Aspirin-induced asthma
    3. Allergen-induced asthma
    4. Intrinsic-specific trigger asthma
        a. 1 and 2 only
        b. 2 and 4 only
        c. 1, 2, and 3 only
        d. 1, 2, 3, and 4

18. Which of the following foods does the manufacturer recommend that montelukast granules be mixed with when given to a child?
    1. Breast milk
    2. Applesauce
    3. Carrots
    4. Rice
        a. 1 and 2 only
        b. 2 and 4 only
        c. 1, 2, and 3 only
        d. 1, 2, 3, and 4

19. Cromolyn prevents the extrusion of granules containing mediators of inflammation to the cell exterior. For this reason, cromolyn is referred to as a:
    a. Goblet cell inhibitor
    b. Nitric oxide stabilizer
    c. Protease inhibitor
    d. Mast cell stabilizer

20. Which of the following is a potent vasodilator that can damage cells and contribute to epithelial damage in asthma?
    a. Neurobinin A
    b. Nitric oxide
    c. Neurobinin B
    d. Neuropeptide

CASE STUDY

Todd is a 3-year-old boy who is in the doctor's office today for evaluation of his asthma. His asthma has been diagnosed as mild to moderate, and he uses a β agonist. After his evaluation, the doctor has decided to put Todd on a medication to help control his asthma. After discussing this with his mother, the doctor sends them to the asthma educator in the office for further consultation.

1. You are the asthma educator; what medication would you recommend for Todd? Why?

2. Because Todd is also receiving a bronchodilator by small volume nebulizer, his mom asks whether a small volume nebulizer can also give the medication, because it would be easiest, given that Todd has difficulty swallowing tablets. What would you tell her?

3. What instruction would you give his mother about how Todd could take this medication?

4. Todd's mom also would like to know whether there is a specific time of the day that Todd should take this medication. What would you tell her?

13 Aerosolized Antiinfective Agents

CHAPTER OUTLINE

Key Terms and Definitions
Clinical Indications for Aerosolized Antiinfective Agents
Inhaled Zanamivir
National Board of Respiratory Care (NBRC) Testing Questions
Case Studies 1 and 2

CHAPTER OBJECTIVES

After answering the following questions, the reader should be able to:

1. Define terms that pertain to aerosolized antiinfective agents
2. Discuss the indications for inhaled antiinfective agents
3. List all available inhaled antiinfective agents used in respiratory therapy
4. Differentiate between the specific antiinfective agent formulations
5. Discuss the route of administration available for the various antiinfective agents
6. Describe the mechanism of action for the various antiinfective agents
7. Recognize side effects for the various antiinfective agents
8. Discuss the use of each antiinfective agent in the treatment of lung disease

KEY TERMS AND DEFINITIONS

Complete the following questions by writing the answer in the space provided.

1. An agent that stops a virus from replicating is called _____.

2. The virus that causes formation of syncytial masses in infected cell structures is _____ _____ _____.

3. An inherited disease of the exocrine glands, affecting the pancreas, respiratory system, and apocrine glands, is called _____. Symptoms usually begin in infancy and are characterized by increased electrolytes in the sweat, chronic respiratory infection, pancreatic insufficiency, and reduced fertility (females) and sterility (males).

4. The pneumonia common among patients with lowered immune system response is _____ _____.

5. An agent that kills a virus is described as _____.

6. A _____ can be defined as an obligate intracellular parasite, containing either DNA or RNA that reproduces by synthesis of subunits within the host cell and causing disease as a consequence of this replication.

CLINICAL INDICATIONS FOR AEROSOLIZED ANTIINFECTIVE AGENTS

7. What is the indication for the following antiinfective agents? Also give the brand name.

   a. Pentamidine: _____, _____

   b. Ribavirin: _____, _____

   c. Tobramycin: _____, _____, _____

   d. Zanamivir: _____, _____

   e. Aztreonam: _____, _____

   f. Palivizumab: _____, _____

8. Pentamidine (NebuPent) is an _____ agent.

9. In patients with acquired immunodeficiency syndrome (AIDS), what is the normal treatment dose and route of pentamidine?

10. What is the name of the nebulizer system recommended for use with pentamidine administration?

11. What is the flow rate used with the Respirgard II nebulizer systems seen in Figure 13-3 in the textbook?

12. For effective nebulization of pentamidine, the mass median diameter (MMD) of particles should be in the range of _____ _____ μm.

13. The most common local side effect from aerosol administration of pentamidine is a(n) _____.

14. When is ribavirin indicated for use in the clinical setting?

15. What is the dose of ribavirin administered by the small-particle aerosol generator (SPAG)-2 nebulizer system?

16. When using a SPAG-2 nebulizer system in line with a mechanical ventilator, what should the respiratory therapist consistently monitor?

17. What is the reason for nearly continuous nebulization of ribavirin?

18. Give one example of a side effect of ribavirin that is associated with the following:

    a. Pulmonary: _____

    b. Cardiovascular: _____

    c. Dermatologic/topical: _____

19. What is the indication for Palivizumab (Synagis)?

20. What is the route of administration and frequency of Palivizumab?

21. Why is aerosolized tobramycin (TOBI) used with patients diagnosed with cystic fibrosis (CF)?

    a. _____

    b. _____

22. True or False: TOBI should be taken before other therapies, including chest physical therapy and bronchodilator therapy, to achieve the greatest airway clearance of secretions.

23. True or False: TOBI can be mixed with dornase alfa to achieve a synergistic effect.

24. Is a specific nebulizer and compressor system recommended for delivery of TOBI? If yes, what is it?

25. What is the dose and frequency for delivery of aerosolized TOBI?

26. What is the clinical use of inhaled aztreonam (Cayston)?

27. What medication should the patient be pretreated with before delivery of Cayston?

28. True of False. Cayston may also be used for patients with CF who are infected with *Burkholderia cepacia*.

INHALED ZANAMIVIR

29. _____ is an antiviral agent approved for use in the treatment of influenza in adults and children more than 5 years of age within the first 2 days of infection.

30. Before treating a patient with an aerosolized antiinfective, what must you do?

31. True or False: A short-acting β agonist can be given to prevent bronchospasm associated with administration of pentamidine.

32. True or False: When administering ribavirin to a child receiving mechanical ventilation, the respiratory therapist should consistently monitor in-line filters for obstruction resulting from drug precipitate.

33. True or False: Before administering aerosolized TOBI, the patient should be instructed that other inhaled medications should be taken.

34. True or False: A patient using zanamivir dry powder inhaler (DPI) should not use a bronchodilator if airway irritation causes bronchospasm.

NATIONAL BOARD OF RESPIRATORY CARE (NBRC) TESTING QUESTIONS

1. Pentamidine is considered to be which of the following?
   a. Antifungal
   b. Antiparasitic
   c. Antiprotozoal
   d. Antibacterial

2. Pentamidine may be administered by which of the following routes of administration?
   1. Oral
   2. Inhalation
   3. IV
   4. Suppository
      a. 1 and 4 only
      b. 2 and 3 only
      c. 1, 2, and 3 only
      d. 1, 2, 3, and 4

3. The only device currently approved by the U.S. Food and Drug Administration for the administration of pentamidine (NebuPent) is which of the following?
   a. SPAG-2
   b. Respirgard II
   c. AeroTech II
   d. Fisoneb

4. Small volume nebulizers (SVNs) used to deliver pentamidine should be equipped with which of the following?
   1. Inspiratory filter
   2. Expiratory filter
   3. One-way valves
   4. Compression generators
      a. 3 and 4 only
      b. 2 and 3 only
      c. 1 and 2 only
      d. 1, 2, and 4 only

5. Ribavirin is classified as which of the following?
   a. Antiprotozoal
   b. Antifungal
   c. Antibacterial
   d. Antiviral

6. Which of the following is the clinical indication for ribavirin?
   a. Prophylactic treatment of *Pneumocystis carinii* pneumonia (PCP)
   b. Treatment of respiratory synctial virus (RSV) infection
   c. Treatment of chronic *Pseudomonas aeruginosa* infection
   d. Treatment of noninfluenza virus infection

7. For effective nebulization of pentamidine, the MMD of particles should be in the range of:
   a. 1 to 2 μm
   b. 3 to 4 μm
   c. 5 to 8 μm
   d. 1 to 10 μm

8. The standard dose of ribavirin administered by the SPAG-2 nebulizer system is:
   a. 10 mg/mL
   b. 20 mg/mL
   c. 30 mg/mL
   d. 35 mg/mL

9. In the northern hemisphere, RSV season runs from:
   a. January to April
   b. January to November
   c. November to April
   d. December to January

10. Which of the following are indications for Cayston use in patients with CF?
    1. To treat influenza type B infections
    2. To treat and prevent early colonization of *P. aeruginosa*
    3. To maintain present lung function
    4. To reduce the rate of deterioration of lung function
       a. 1 and 2 only
       b. 1 and 3 only
       c. 2, 3, and 4 only
       d. 1, 2, 3, and 4

11. Which of the following nebulizers is recommended for use to administer TOBI?
    a. SPAG-2
    b. Respirgard II
    c. Aerojet III
    d. PARI LC Plus

12. In what other disease can TOBI be used to treat *P. aeruginosa* infections?
    a. RSV
    b. Bronchiolitis
    c. Congenital heart disease
    d. No other diseases at this time

13. Which of the following statements is *true* regarding TOBI?
    a. Chest physical therapy should be administered as the patient is breathing TOBI.
    b. Dornase alfa may be mixed with TOBI to achieve a synergistic effect.
    c. TOBI should be administered after administration of all other therapy or medications.
    d. TOBI should be mixed with a short-acting β agonist to prevent bronchospasm.

14. A treatment dose of _____ mg of zanamivir is recommended for influenza infection.
    a. 5
    b. 10
    c. 20
    d. 200

15. Which of the following is the reason that ribavirin is administered for 12 to 18 hours per day for the treatment of RSV?
    a. A large quantity of drug rainout occurs because of the large particles formed from the SPAG-2 device.
    b. The powder creates increased rainout of the drug within the SPAG-2 nebulizer system.
    c. The drug has a short half-life in respiratory secretions.
    d. The liver metabolizes the drug quickly.

16. During the short-term respiratory care of a patient receiving TOBI, what assessments should occur?
    1. Monitor lung function
    2. Assess for improvement in weight
    3. Evaluate changes in hearing
    4. Monitor for signs of RSV
        a. 1 and 3 only
        b. 2 and 4 only
        c. 1, 2, and 3 only
        d. 2, 3, and 4 only

17. What is a clinical indication for the use of aztreonam (Cayston)?
    a. Forced expiratory volume at 1 second (FEV_1) lower than 20%
    b. *Pseudomonas aeruginosa* colonization
    c. *Staphylococcus aureus* colonization
    d. *Burkholderia cepacia* colonization

18. Zanamivir (Relenza) is approved for children:
    a. Less than 1 year of age
    b. 2 to 3 years of age
    c. Greater than 5 years of age
    d. Greater than 12 years of age

19. Which of the following statements is *true* regarding administration of ribavirin in children?
    a. It should be administered immediately on diagnosis of routine RSV infection.
    b. It should be administered after 3 days of bronchodilator treatments have not been effective.
    c. It may be considered for life-threatening RSV infection.
    d. It should be considered only for children less than 6 months of age.

20. Oseltamivir phosphate (Tamiflu) has an off-label use for:
    a. Mild RSV
    b. H1N1 (swine flu)
    c. Bronchiolitis in infants with a history of prematurity
    d. RSV in infants with a history of congenital heart disease

CASE STUDY 1

Your patient, who was diagnosed with human immunodeficiency virus (HIV) in 1994, presents with a $CD4^+$ cell count of $100/mm^3$, fever, shaking, chills, and productive cough. He has had PCP once before this admission. His diagnosis is PCP, and his physician has ordered pentamidine (NebuPent) treatments four times daily for treatment. As you do your pretreatment assessment, the patient tells you that he has previously been given pentamidine and that "It makes me cough pretty much throughout the whole treatment."

1. What do you recommend?

As a favor to you, one of your colleagues begins this treatment, using an SVN.

2. Should your colleague be using an SVN to administer pentamidine?

3. Other than using the Respirgard II, what precautions should you take to minimize your exposure to the pentamidine?

   a. _____

   b. _____

   c. _____

4. What adverse effects are you likeliest to suffer as a result of exposure to pentamidine?

CASE STUDY 2

Jeremy is a 7-year-old boy who has been in the hospital for the past 3 days for treatment of CF. He is being discharged, and his physician has ordered TOBI to be added to his pulmonary hygiene routine. Because this is the first time Jeremy will be taking TOBI, his parents have some questions. The physician has asked the respiratory therapist to meet with Jeremy and his parents to discuss the use of TOBI and to answer any other questions.

1. One of the first questions Jeremy's parents ask is: "What is TOBI, and why is he getting this drug?"

2. The next question is: "How much drug is Jeremy going to receive, and how often will he need to take it?"

3. His parents then ask: "Can this medication be nebulized in the same equipment that he is using for his dornase alpha and albuterol?"

4. His mother states: "Currently Jeremy takes his aerosolized medications with his Vest treatment. Can he just add the TOBI to his other medications as he does his Vest treatment? This really helps him in the morning to save time when he is getting ready to go to school."

5. His dad asks: "Does TOBI have any side effects?"

6. Jeremy and his parents are concerned about the voice alteration: "Is there anything that can be done to minimize it or prevent this from occurring?"

14 Antimicrobial Agents

CHAPTER OUTLINE

Key Terms and Definitions
Principles of Antimicrobial Therapy
    Identification of the Pathogen
    Susceptibility Testing and Resistance
    Host Factors
    Pharmacodynamics and Antimicrobial Combinations
Monitoring Response to Therapy
Antibiotics
Antiviral Agents
National Board of Respiratory Care (NBRC) Testing Questions
Case Studies 1 and 2

CHAPTER OBJECTIVES

After answering the following questions, the reader should be able to:

1. Define terms that pertain to antimicrobial agents
2. Define *antibiotic*
3. Describe the process involved in bacterial susceptibility testing
4. Discuss possible outcomes of antimicrobial combinations
5. List the various classes of the penicillins
6. List the various classes of the cephalosporins
7. Recognize similarities between members of the macrolides, azalides, and ketolides
8. Recognize similarities between members of the fluoroquinolones
9. List four mechanisms of action of antibacterials
10. List five commonly used antimycobacterials
11. Describe the commonly used azole antifungals and how they differ in spectrum of activity
12. Discuss similarities between members of the echinocandins
13. Describe the mechanism of action of the antiretrovirals

KEY TERMS AND DEFINITIONS

Complete the following by writing the answer in the space provided.

1. Both natural and synthetic compounds that either inhibit or kill microorganisms are called _____.

2. The term _____ describes when the combined effect of two antimicrobials is greater than their added effects.

3. Natural compounds that produced by microorganisms that either inhibit or kill other microorganisms, are called _____.

4. The term _____ describes when the effect of a combination of two antimicrobials is lower than the effect expected from either agent alone.

PRINCIPLES OF ANTIMICROBIAL THERAPY

5. List four factors that must be considered before choosing an antimicrobial agent.

   a. _____

   b. _____

   c. _____

   d. _____

Identification of the Pathogen

6. What steps would need to be taken to identify the pathogen causing infection in a patient?

7. As a respiratory therapist, what is likely the most common specimen you will collect for culture?

8. The simplest and most common preparation by which to identify bacteria is the _____ _____.

9. Gram-positive bacteria stain _____ and gram-negative bacteria stain _____.

10. What is responsible for the difference in staining in a Gram stain?

11. *Mycobacterium tuberculosis* requires a(n) _____-_____ stain to penetrate its waxlike cell wall.

12. Match the following common pathogens with their associated respiratory infection(s) in the adult.

    1. _____ Sinusitis
    2. _____ Community-acquired pneumonia (CAP)
    3. _____ Hospital-acquired pneumonia
    4. _____ Acute bronchitis
    5. _____ Cystic fibrosis (CF)

    a. *Staphylococcus aureus*
    b. *Mycoplasma pneumoniae*
    c. *Staphylococcus pneumoniae*
    d. *Haemophilus influenzae*
    e. *Streptococcus pneumoniae*

Susceptibility Testing and Resistance

13. Explain the *zone of inhibition* as it relates to susceptibility testing.

Host Factors

14. Describe a clinical situation where a patient may fail to respond to antimicrobial therapy.

15. Describe a clinical situation that may require adjustment of an antimicrobial drug dosage schedule.

16. Bactericidal drugs _____ bacteria, whereas bacteriostatic drugs _____ growth of bacteria.

Pharmacodynamics and Antimicrobial Combinations

17. _____ the phenomenon in which bacterial growth is inhibited even after the drug level drops below detectable levels.

18. When two or more classes of antimicrobials are combined, they should act _____, not antagonistically.

MONITORING RESPONSE TO THERAPY

19. Although certain laboratory parameters can be monitored to assess the efficacy of an antimicrobial regimen, response to therapy is best measured by _____ _____.

ANTIBIOTICS

20. Penicillins and cephalosporins exert their pharmacologic activity by inhibiting _____ _____ synthesis.

21. Cephalosporins inhibit _____ _____ _____ in a manner similar to penicillin.

22. Carbapenems are _____-_____ antibiotics effective against gram-positive and gram-negative bacteria.

23. True or False: The monobactam aztreonam is active only against gram-negative aerobic bacilli such as *Pseudomonas aeruginosa*.

24. List two examples of aminoglycosides that are used in the treatment of cystic fibrosis (CF).
    a. _____
    b. _____

25. List three aminoglycosides that are used in the treatment of ventilator-associated pneumonia (VAP).
    a. _____
    b. _____
    c. _____

26. _____ broad-spectrum antibiotics that are used in both pulmonary and systemic infections and are effective for treatment of diseases such as Rocky Mountain spotted fever, Lyme disease, and others.

27. Tetracyclines inhibit _____ _____, resulting in a bacteriostatic effect.

28. The drug of choice for *Legionella* bacteria is _____.

29. Vancomycin is useful for the treatment of infections caused by _____-_____ _____ _____.

30. What is one explanation for the increase in number of tuberculosis (TB) cases since 2000?

31. Patients with suspected TB should remain in their hospital room until one of the following three criteria is met. List all three.

    a. _____

    b. _____

    c. _____

32. Drug treatment for tuberculosis consists of multiple antibiotics for _____ to _____ months.

33. *M. tuberculosis* is spread by _____.

34. The incidence of fungal infections has increased dramatically, with _____ species now the fourth most commonly isolated bloodstream pathogen.

35. Fungal infections have increased over the past years because of:

    a. _____

    b. _____

    c. _____

ANTIVIRAL AGENTS

36. Antiviral agents (excluding antiretrovirals) mimic nucleosides and inhibit _____ _____ _____.

NATIONAL BOARD OF RESPIRATORY CARE (NBRC) TESTING QUESTIONS

1. The simplest and most common preparation by which to identify bacteria is the:
   a. Acid-fast stain
   b. Gram stain
   c. Ziehl-Neelsen smear
   d. Agar plate count

2. Gram-positive bacteria stain _____, using the Gram stain method.
   a. Purple
   b. Red
   c. Pink
   d. Orange

3. An acid-fast stain is used to identify:
   a. *P. aeruginosa*
   b. *S. pneumoniae*
   c. *Candida* species
   d. *M. tuberculosis*

4. Which of the following common pathogens cause CAP?
   a. *S. aureus*
   b. *Mycobacterium pneumoniae*
   c. *P. aeruginosa*
   d. *H. influenzae*

5. A bacteriostatic drug is one that:
   a. Kills bacteria
   b. Inhibits bacterial growth
   c. Terminates replication
   d. Interferes with DNA replication

6. Although certain laboratory parameters can be monitored to assess efficacy of an antimicrobial regimen, response to therapy is best measured by:
   a. The number of antibiotics the patient is currently taking
   b. The strength of antibiotics the patient is currently taking
   c. The number of days the patient has been taking antibiotics
   d. Clinical assessment

7. Penicillins and cephalosporins exert their pharmacologic activity by inhibiting:
   a. Cell wall synthesis
   b. DNA replication
   c. RNA replication
   d. Viral replication

8. Broad-spectrum antibiotics are effective against:
   1. Viral infections
   2. Fungal infections
   3. Gram-positive infections
   4. Gram-negative infections
      a. 1 and 2 only
      b. 3 and 4 only
      c. 1, 2, and 4 only
      d. 1, 2, 3, and 4

9. Which of the following aminoglycosides is used to treat CF?
   1. Amikacin
   2. Cephalosporins
   3. Tobramycin
   4. Tetracycline
      a. 1 and 2 only
      b. 1 and 3 only
      c. 3 and 4 only
      d. 1, 2, and 3 only

10. Which of the following drugs is used in the treatment of VAP?
    a. Erythromycin
    b. Tetracycline
    c. Fluoroquinolones
    d. Gentamicin

11. The drug of choice for *Legionella* bacteria is:
    a. Tetracycline
    b. Erythromycin
    c. Penicillin
    d. Gentamicin

12. Methicillin-resistant *S. aureus* (MRSA) is best treated with which of the following?
    a. Vancomycin
    b. Clindamycin
    c. Erythromycin
    d. Gentamicin

13. A patient suspected of having TB should remain in an isolation room until which of the following criteria is met?
    a. The patient is determined not to have TB.
    b. The patient has been pharmacologically treated for 5 days.
    c. The patient has three sputum samples obtained over a 3-day period.
    d. The patient no longer needs protective barriers, such as masks.

14. Drug treatment for tuberculosis consists of multiple antibiotics for:
    a. 5 to 7 days
    b. 12 to 15 days
    c. 1 to 2 months
    d. 6 to 12 months

15. Nosocomial transmission can be prevented by placing patients with suspected or confirmed tuberculosis in:
    a. Contact isolation
    b. Reverse isolation
    c. Respiratory isolation
    d. MRSA contact isolation

16. Initial therapy for treatment of TB involves a combination of which of the following medications?
    1. Isoniazid
    2. Pyrazinamide
    3. Rifampin
    4. Ethambutol
        a. 1 and 3 only
        b. 2 and 4 only
        c. 1, 2, and 4 only
        d. 1, 2, 3, and 4

17. Which of the following pathogens are commonly responsible for CAP?
    1. *S. pneumoniae*
    2. *H. influenzae*
    3. *M. pneumoniae*
    4. *Legionella pneumophila*
        a. 1 and 2 only
        b. 3 and 4 only
        c. 1, 3, and 4 only
        d. 1, 2, 3, and 4

18. A sputum culture has returned and shows gram-negative bacilli (rods) present. This result would indicate:
    a. Colonization
    b. Hospital-acquired pneumonia
    c. Nosocomial pneumonia
    d. Aspiration pneumonia

19. Incidence of fungal infections has increased, and the most common species responsible for fungal infections is:
    a. *Scedosporium*
    b. *Candida*
    c. *Aspergillus*
    d. *Fusarium*

20. Which of the following are viral infections that would be treated with antiviral medications?
    1. Herpes simplex 1
    2. Herpes zoster
    3. Varicella-zoster
    4. Cytomegalovirus
        a. 1 and 3 only
        b. 2 and 4 only
        c. 1, 3, and 4 only
        d. 1, 2, 3 and 4

CASE STUDY 1

Mr. Green lives in a homeless shelter in downtown Atlanta; he moved there from New Orleans after Hurricane Katrina. He has developed symptoms including a productive cough with blood-tinged sputum, chills, and sweating. He went to a local hospital emergency department, where he is diagnosed with TB.

1. What treatment regimen should be recommended for him?

2. Mr. Green has been admitted to the hospital. To prevent nosocomial transmission of TB, what would you suggest to provide respiratory isolation of this patient?

3. How long will Mr. Green have to remain in respiratory isolation?

4. What other measures should be recommended to health care employees entering Mr. Green's room that will help prevent the spread of *M. tuberculosis* by aerosolization?

CASE STUDY 2

Mrs. Palermo has been admitted to the hospital and is diagnosed with pneumonia. Physical assessment reveals a temperature of 38.5° C, a nonproductive cough, bibasilar crackles, and expiratory wheezing in all lung fields. Laboratory test results show an elevated white blood count (WBC). The respiratory therapist has been contacted to give breathing treatments and obtain a sputum sample for culture.

1. Many patients do not produce sputum with pneumonia, so what are common pathogens that cause pneumonia that may be considered for antibiotic therapy before obtaining a culture?

2. In the meantime, while waiting for a sputum sample for culture, what can be done to begin treating Mrs. Palermo's pneumonia?

3. After several breathing treatments, the patient produces enough sputum for culture. Analysis shows the patient to have an *S. pneumoniae* infection. What antibiotic could be helpful for this pathogen?

After several days of treatments, the patient's symptoms improve and WBC normalizes. The patient is sent home with several medications, including a 10-day supply of antibiotics, and is instructed to take all the medication. She also has an appointment see her primary care physician in 2 weeks. Five days after being discharged from the hospital, Mrs. Palermo calls her primary care physician and explains that her temperature has returned, she is coughing and producing sputum, and she is feeling similar to when she entered the hospital.

4. What would you recommend asking the patient to help determine why her symptoms have returned?

15 Cold and Cough Agents

CHAPTER OUTLINE

Key Terms and Definitions
Sympathomimetic (Adrenergic) Decongestants
Antihistamine Agents
Expectorants
Cough Suppressants (Antitussives)
Cold Compounds: Treating a Cold
National Board of Respiratory Care (NBRC) Testing Questions
Case Studies 1 and 2

CHAPTER OBJECTIVES

After answering the following questions, the reader should be able to:

1. Define key terms that pertain to cold and cough agents
2. Differentiate between the common cold and the flu
3. Differentiate between the specific types of cold and cough agents
4. Discuss the mode of action for each specific cold and cough agent

KEY TERMS AND DEFINITIONS

Complete the following by writing the answer in the space provided.

1. Drugs that reduce the effects mediated by histamine, a chemical released by the body during allergic reactions, are called _____.

2. The _____ is a nonbacterial infection, characterized by a rapid onset of symptoms that include fever, headache, and fatigue.

3. Agents that increase the production and therefore presumably the clearance of mucus secretions in the respiratory tract, such as guaifenesin, are called _____ _____.

4. The best _____, especially with colds, is plain water and juices; caffeinated beverages, such as tea or colas, and beer or other alcoholic mixtures should be avoided.

5. A nonbacterial respiratory tract infection, characterized by malaise and a runny nose, is called a(n) _____ _____.

6. Agents that facilitate removal of mucus by a lysing or mucolytic action, such as dornase alfa, are called _____ _____.

7. Drugs that suppress the cough reflex, and are useful in the presence of an irritating, persistent, nonproductive cough, are called _____.

8. Match the following signs and symptoms of the common cold and influenza.

9. Drugs that can cause rebound congestion if taken longer than a day and mimic the effects of the sympathetic nervous system are _____.

   1. _____ Fever
   2. _____ No chills present
   3. _____ Headache
   4. _____ Nonproductive cough
   5. _____ Nasal congestion (common)
   6. _____ Early and severe fatigue
   7. _____ Sore throat (common)

   a. Cold
   b. Influenza

10. List four classes of drugs available to treat the common cold:

    a. _____
    b. _____
    c. _____
    d. _____

11. List the indications for each of the four classes listed in question 10.

    a. _____
    b. _____
    c. _____
    d. _____

SYMPATHOMIMETIC (ADRENERGIC) DECONGESTANTS

12. How long should adrenergic nasal sprays be used? Explain why.

13. Topical sympathomimetic _____ sprays or drops produce results faster than oral applications.

ANTIHISTAMINE AGENTS

14. Where are the following receptors located, and what does stimulation of each result in?

    a. H_1: _____
    b. H_2: _____
    c. H_3: _____

15. What are three effects of antihistamines?

    a. _____
    b. _____
    c. _____

16. The anticholinergic effect of first-generation H_1 receptor cold medications contributes to _____ _____ drying.

EXPECTORANTS

17. What are three ways stimulant expectorants work?

    a. _____

    b. _____

    c. _____

18. The best expectorant for a simple cold is _____.

19. How do bland aerosols of saline increase sputum volume?

    a. _____

    b. _____

COUGH SUPPRESSANTS (ANTITUSSIVES)

20. List a situation in which the use of antitussives would not be indicated.

21. A common narcotic cough suppressant is _____.

COLD COMPOUNDS: TREATING A COLD

Complete the following by writing the undesirable effects of each category of ingredient in the space provided.

22. Sympathomimetics

    a. _____

    b. _____

    c. _____

23. Antihistamines

    a. _____

    b. _____

    c. _____

24. Expectorants

    a. _____

25. Antitussives

    a. _____

NATIONAL BOARD OF RESPIRATORY CARE (NBRC) TESTING QUESTIONS

1. Which of the following agents is useful in the presence of an irritating, persistent, nonproductive cough?
   a. Antitussive
   b. Expectorant
   c. Mucolytic expectorant
   d. Sympathomimetic

2. Which of the following symptoms is *not* associated with the flu?
   a. Fever
   b. Sore throat
   c. Fatigue
   d. Headache

3. An antihistamine used to treat a common cold is intended to:
   a. Decongest
   b. Suppress the cough reflex
   c. Dry secretions
   d. Increase mucus clearance

4. Which of the following is *false* concerning the common cold?
   a. It is a nonbacterial respiratory tract infection.
   b. It is characterized by a runny nose.
   c. Nasal congestion is rare.
   d. Sneezing and sore throat are present.

5. An agent that increases the production and clearance of mucus secretions in the respiratory tract is called a(n):
   a. Antihistamine
   b. Antitussive
   c. Mucolytic expectorant
   d. Stimulant expectorant

6. Classes of drugs that are available to treat the common cold include:
   1. Sympathomimetics
   2. Antihistamines
   3. Expectorants
   4. Antitussives
      a. 1 and 2 only
      b. 2 and 3 only
      c. 1, 3, and 4 only
      d. 1, 2, 3, and 4

7. An alternative to antihistamines for rhinorrhea in a cold is the anticholinergic nasal spray:
   a. Spiriva
   b. Combivent
   c. Atrovent
   d. DuoNeb

8. Nasal decongestion is achieved by sympathomimetics by stimulation of which receptor?
   a. β_1
   b. β_2
   c. α
   d. H_1

9. The common cold is usually _____ in origin.
   a. Bacterial
   b. Viral
   c. Fungal
   d. Allergenic

10. Which of the following is associated with "rebound congestion" concerning oral administration of sympathomimetic decongestants?
    a. Slower onset of action
    b. Better decongestion
    c. Increased systemic side effects
    d. Overuse of these agents

11. Which of the following classes of effects applies or apply to antihistamines?
    1. Antihistaminic
    2. Sedative
    3. Anticholinergic
    4. Sympathomimetic
       a. 4
       b. 2 and 3
       c. 1, 2, and 3
       d. 1, 3, and 4

12. The anticholinergic effect of antihistamines on the upper airway results in:
    a. Bronchoconstriction
    b. Capillary leakage
    c. Drying
    d. Increased mucus production

13. Which of the following is recommended as being safe and effective as an expectorant?
    a. Terpin hydrate
    b. Guaifenesin
    c. Glycerol
    d. Iodine

14. The best expectorant for a cold is:
    a. Water
    b. Terpin hydrate
    c. Guaifenesin
    d. Glycerol

15. Which of the following side effects is most associated with an antihistamine?
    a. Tremor
    b. Drowsiness
    c. Hypertension
    d. Tachycardia

16. Which of the following is best for a patient who has a nonproductive, irritating, dry, hacking cough?
    a. Expectorant
    b. Antihistamine
    c. Cough suppressant
    d. Sympathetic stimulant

17. You see an ad on television for a cold remedy that contains dextromethorphan. You call your spouse, who is at the store, and tell them to get:
    a. Vicks 44 cough relief
    b. Robitussin
    c. Sudafed
    d. Claritin

18. Which of the following Robitussin medications would you want to avoid during the day while working or driving?
    a. Robitussin cold and cough
    b. Robitussin DAC
    c. Robitussin Cough and Allergy
    d. Robitussin Sneeze and Wheeze

19. A rational approach to surviving colds and preventing spread of rhinovirus is:
    1. Yearly flu shot
    2. Antibiotics
    3. Fluids
    4. Rest
        a. 1 and 2
        b. 2 and 4
        c. 3 and 4
        d. 2, 3, and 4

20. If a patient has cardiovascular problems and is using a decongestant, which of the following should be monitored for this patient?
    1. Blood pressure
    2. Oxygen saturation
    3. Temperature
    4. Heart rate
        a. 2 and 3
        b. 2 and 4
        c. 1, 2, and 4
        d. 2, 3, and 4

CASE STUDY 1

Your parents are away on a cruise and left you babysitting your little brother during spring break. Over the past few days, he has developed a runny nose, is sneezing, and says he feels "icky." You take his temperature and it is 98.8° F.

1. What is the most likely diagnosis?

2. What treatment would help him the most at present?

3. Being a good respiratory therapist, you anticipate that he may develop a cough that is dry and nonproductive, even though his temperature remains normal. You ask yourself: "Is there anything in his treatment regimen that can be changed so that I won't have to take him to the doctor?"

CASE STUDY 2

You are a respiratory therapist working for a home care company. You are visiting a patient, Mrs. Fields, to check on some equipment she is renting. While you are there, she tells you that she doesn't feel well. She says she felt fine 2 days ago, but today she has a nonproductive cough that keeps her awake at night, chills, headache, no energy, and aching muscles. She asks: "Do you think I have a cold?"

1. Based on her description of symptoms, what would you tell her?

2. What infectious agent may have caused this illness?

3. She says that the worst part about this illness is a dry, hacking, nonproductive cough that keeps her awake at night. She asks you whether there is something she can take that would stop her coughing so she can sleep. What would you tell her?

4. What precaution would you want to tell Mrs. Fields about taking this medication during the daytime?

16 Selected Agents of Pulmonary Value

CHAPTER OUTLINE

Key Terms and Definitions
National Board of Respiratory Care (NBRC) Testing Questions
Case Studies 1 and 2

CHAPTER OBJECTIVES

After answering the following questions, the reader should be able to:

1. Define key terms and definitions pertaining to selected agents of pulmonary value
2. Discuss the indication for α_1-proteinase inhibitor
3. Recognize α_1-proteinase inhibitor deficiency in a patient
4. List the α_1-proteinase inhibitors that are available
5. List three types of formulations for nicotine replacement
6. Recognize the advantages and disadvantages of nicotine replacement
7. Discuss the indication for nitric oxide
8. Describe the effect of inhaled nitric oxide on a patient
9. List the two toxic products of nitric oxide
10. List the two inhaled prostacyclin analogs available in the United States

KEY TERMS AND DEFINITIONS

Match the following definitions with their terms.

1. _____ α_1-Proteinase inhibitor (API) has altered electrophoretic properties and lower-than-normal serum concentrations

2. _____ Also known as α_1-*proteinase inhibitor*, this inhibitor of trypsin may be deficient in patients with emphysema

3. _____ Undetectable API levels in the serum

4. _____ API is present in normal amounts, but does not function normally

5. _____ Individual has normal serum levels of API

a. α_1-Antitrypsin (α_1-AT)
b. API deficient
c. API dysfunctional
d. API normal
e. API null

6. How is α_1-AT (Prolastin) prepared?

7. α_1-AT deficiency, similar to cystic fibrosis, is an _____ _____ disorder.

8. The enzyme neutrophil elastase, which can destroy alveolar walls, is held in check by _____.

9. Explain the pathogenesis of emphysema caused by α_1-AT deficiency.

10. For individuals with congenital deficiency of API, with clinically demonstrable panacinar emphysema, _____ _____ _____ is indicated as long-term replacement therapy.

11. True or False: Given the nature of the disease and the action of the drugs, α_1-AT proteinase-inhibiting drugs cannot reverse damage or improve lung function.

12. Indicate whether the following statements are either *True* or *False* concerning assessment of α_1-AT replacement therapy.
    a. True or False: Overall pulmonary health should be assessed, based on frequency and severity of respiratory infections, cough, sputum production if present, and hospitalization rate.
    b. True or False: Pulmonary function testing of flow rates is used to monitor the degree of airflow obstruction for short-term use of the drug.

13. Nicotine stimulates the _____ receptors at the autonomic ganglia of both the sympathetic and parasympathetic nervous systems.

14. List seven physical symptoms a patient may experience during nicotine withdrawal.
    a. _____
    b. _____
    c. _____
    d. _____
    e. _____
    f. _____
    g. _____

15. List five forms of nicotine replacement.
    a. _____
    b. _____
    c. _____
    d. _____
    e. _____

16. What is the indication for nicotine replacement therapy? Who benefits most from therapy?

17. Explain why the nicotine inhaler may be preferred to gum and nasal spray.

18. _____ is an antidepressant found in Wellbutrin; it is also a nonnicotine aid to smoking cessation.

19. Chantix is used to block receptors for _____, thus reducing the sensation produced by smoking.

20. _____ is an antihypertensive agent that has been prescribed to reduce symptoms of opioid and alcohol withdrawal.

21. Nitric oxide (NO) is a gas that is inhaled to cause selective _____ vasodilation.

22. Indications for inhaled nitric oxide (INO) are neonates with a gestational age of _____ weeks with _____ respiratory failure associated with clinical evidence of _____ hypertension.

23. The recommended dosage of INO is _____ ppm.

24. Administration of INO at more than the recommended dose can cause increased levels of _____ _____ and _____.

25. According to the American Academy of Pediatrics, sample gas for analysis should be drawn _____ the wye adaptor, proximal to the patient.

26. True or False: Blood methemoglobin levels should be drawn every other day.

27. True or False: Weaning from NO should be gradual to prevent arterial desaturation and pulmonary hypertension.

28. True or False: The dose of NO should always start at 40 ppm and can be increased to 80 ppm if no clinical signs of pulmonary vasodilation occur.

29. True or False: Because INO has a short half-life, as soon as the INO is discontinued, pulmonary vasodilation ends.

30. Because of the rapid deactivation of NO, the result of its binding to hemoglobin, NO is a _____ pulmonary vasodilator.

31. True or False: The higher the fraction of inspired oxygen (F_iO_2), the greater the amount of oxidation of NO to NO_2.

32. INO becomes inactive when it enters the red blood cell and attaches to _____.

33. Some endogenous NO is exhaled from the lungs after being converted to _____ within the red blood cells.

34. Improvement of arterial oxygen pressure (Pa_{O_2}) with INO results from dilation of pulmonary blood vessels and improved _____ _____ matching.

35. NO is administered to an infant receiving _____ _____.

36. Preductal and postductal shunting can be monitoring during NO delivery by monitoring the _____.

37. Ventavis dilates _____ and _____ vascular beds when given via inhalation.

38. What two aerosol delivery systems are recommended for administration of Ventavis?

    a. _____

    b. _____

39. In patients with chronic obstructive pulmonary disease (COPD) receiving Ventavis, pretreatment with a _____ _____ may be beneficial to prevent bronchospasm.

40. Tyvaso is an inhaled prostacyclin vasodilator for the treatment of _____ _____.

41. Tyvaso should not be used in patients _____ years of age.

42. During administration of Tyvaso, to assess if the patient develops bronchospasm, _____ _____ should be performed during therapy.

NATIONAL BOARD OF RESPIRATORY CARE (NBRC) TESTING QUESTIONS

1. What type of disorder is α_1-AT deficiency?
   a. Autosomal recessive
   b. Disomonal
   c. Trisomy 13
   d. XY recessive

2. Which statement is *true* regarding α_1-AT deficiency?
   a. It is generally seen at a later age, as a result of smoking.
   b. It is caused by excessive exposure to asbestos at an early age.
   c. It develops at an early age among people without cause (smoking, relevant work history).
   d. It develops predominantly in men more than 65 years of age with a history of exposure to wood dust.

3. Which of the following are signs of high physical addiction/dependence on nicotine?
   1. Smokes more than 15 cigarettes per day
   2. Smokes within 30 minutes of rising from bed
   3. Smokes even when bedridden from illness
   4. Smokes more frequently in the morning
      a. 1 and 4 only
      b. 1 and 3 only
      c. 1, 2, and 3 only
      d. 1, 2, 3, and 4

4. What is the purpose of nicotine replacement therapy?
   a. To reduce the number of cigarettes smoked by a patient
   b. To reduce the food cravings of a smoking patient who is cutting down on the number of cigarettes smoked per day
   c. To replace the nicotine lost with smoking cessation
   d. To help eliminate nicotine from the body during weaning from cigarette smoking

5. Which of the following methods of administering nicotine would simulate a cigarette and give oral gratification?
   a. Nicotine gum
   b. Nicotine nasal spray
   c. Nicotine patch
   d. Nicotine inhaler

6. Bupropion (Zyban) contains which of the following?
   1. Nonnicotine agent to help reduce smoking
   2. Antidepressant
   3. Analgesic
   4. Nicotine
      a. 1 and 2 only
      b. 2 and 3 only
      c. 1 and 3 only
      d. 1, 2, and 3 only

7. Before prescribing varenicline (Chantix) to a patient who is currently smoking, you should have the patient set a quit date and start the medication _____ week(s) before this date.
   a. 1
   b. 2
   c. 3
   d. 4

8. The indication for INO is for neonates with a gestational age of:
   a. Greater than 34 weeks
   b. Greater than 24 weeks
   c. Less than 27 weeks
   d. Less than 31 weeks

9. INO is considered to be a selective pulmonary artery vasodilator because:
   a. It is inhaled
   b. The nitric oxide rapidly deactivates once it attaches to hemoglobin
   c. A large dose is administered and the oxygen concentration is high
   d. It converts to nitrogen dioxide, which remains in the lung

10. The recommended dose of INO is:
    a. 80 ppm
    b. 60 ppm
    c. 40 ppm
    d. 20 ppm

11. Administration of NO at more than the recommended levels can increase levels of:
    1. Methemoglobin
    2. Nitrogen dioxide
    3. Sulfhemoglobin
    4. Nitrohemoglobin
       a. 1 and 2 only
       b. 2 and 3 only
       c. 1, 3, and 4 only
       d. 2 and 4 only

12. Approximately _____% of smokers have the genetic substrate resulting in some degree of nicotine addiction.
    a. 10%
    b. 40%
    c. 60%
    d. 90%

13. Use of bupropion is associated with a dose-dependent risk of:
    a. Bronchospasm
    b. Excessive secretions in lower airway
    c. Seizure
    d. Pulmonary artery vasoconstriction

14. Nicotine replacement therapy should be carefully weighed in patients with:
    a. Diabetes type 2
    b. Diabetes type 1
    c. Cardiovascular disease
    d. Asthma

15. According to the American Academy of Pediatrics, sampling of gas containing NO for analysis of a patient on mechanical ventilation should take place:
    a. On the inspiratory side of the patient circuit, where INO first enters the circuit
    b. On the expiratory side of the patient circuit
    c. Before the wye adaptor, proximal to the patient
    d. On the expiratory side of the patient circuit, just before the exhalation valve of the ventilator

16. Which of the following are indications for NO therapy for neonates?
    1. Hypoxic respiratory failure
    2. Lung hypoplasia
    3. Immature lungs and deficient surfactant
    4. Pulmonary hypertension
        a. 1 and 3 only
        b. 2 and 3 only
        c. 1 and 4 only
        d. 1, 3, and 4 only

17. NO is administered to an infant through which of the following?
    a. Nonrebreather mask
    b. High-flow nasal cannula
    c. Mechanical ventilation
    d. Bubble CPAP system

18. Preductal and postductal shunting can be monitored during NO delivery by monitoring which of the following?
    a. Capillary blood gases
    b. Umbilical venous blood gases
    c. Scalp venous blood gases
    d. Pulse oximetry measurement

19. Which of the following aerosol delivery systems is recommended for administration of iloprost (Ventavis)?
    a. Aerogen vibrating mesh
    b. Misty Neb
    c. Prodose ADD system
    d. MicroNeb

20. Prostinil (Tyvaso) is an inhaled prostacyclin vasodilator for the treatment of which of the following?
    a. Pulmonary hypertension
    b. Systemic hypotension
    c. Atrial fibrillation with associated systemic hypotension
    d. Premature ventricular contractions (more than six per minute) with pulmonary hypotension

CASE STUDY 1

You are conducting a smoking cessation class at a local pulmonary rehabilitation clinic. One of the participants is the president of a local university. Because she is new to the class, you interview her to obtain a smoking history and to see whether she has a high physical addiction to nicotine. Her history indicates the following:

She works an average of 60 hours per week and is widely known throughout her community.
She feels she has a high level of stress.
She smokes a pack a day.
She lights her first cigarette within 30 minutes of rising from bed in the morning.
Her smoking occurs mostly in the morning, especially on her one and one-half hour commute to the university.
Even though her campus is smoke free, she admits to slipping out from her office to smoke.

1. Based on her interview, does she have a physical addiction to nicotine?

2. She asks you to recommend the smoking cessation method that would best suit her lifestyle. What would you recommend?

3. After some use of the transdermal patch, she complains that she has skin irritation where she places the patch each day. What would you recommend?

4. Your patient is a heavy smoker (approximately 20 cigarettes a day). What size patch (in milligrams) would be recommended for her level of smoking?

5. After 2 weeks on the transdermal patch, she complains of feeling depressed and feels she cannot continue with the smoking cessation program. What would you suggest?

CASE STUDY 2

A 35-week gestational age infant is currently intubated and receiving mechanical ventilation with an FiO_2 of 1.0 with a resulting SpO_2 of 80%. Echocardiography has been performed and indicates the presence of pulmonary hypertension. The decision has been made to begin *INOmax* therapy inline through the ventilator.

1. What is the recommended initial starting dose of NO?

2. The nurse is concerned about the newborn's systemic blood pressure during delivery of NO, because the baby's blood pressure is currently low. How would you respond to this concern?

3. After 20 minutes, the infant's Spo_2 has increased to 95%. What does this indicate that is occurring in the lungs?

4. A measurement of NO shows it to be 1%. Is this going to be a concern for the formation of methemoglobin?

The infant has now been on *INOmax* for 2 days. Currently, the infant is receiving 18 ppm, and the Fio_2 is 0.60 and Spo_2 is 94%. An order has been written to continue decreasing the NO in increments of 2 ppm. After the NO is decreased to 16 ppm, the Spo_2 drops to 83%.

5. a. Why could this have occurred?

   b. What should be done to increase the Spo_2?

6. What formula could be used to evaluate the relationships among mean airway pressure of the ventilator, ventilator Fio_2, and Pao_2?

17 Neonatal and Pediatric Aerosolized Drug Therapy

CHAPTER OUTLINE

Key Terms and Definitions
Introduction
Unlabeled Use of Drugs in Neonatal and Pediatric Patients
Factors Affecting Neonatal and Pediatric Aerosol Drug Delivery
Clinical Response to Aerosolized Drugs in Neonatal and Pediatric Patients
Selection of Delivery Devices
Compliance and Cooperation During Aerosol Therapy
Aerosol Administration in Intubated Neonatal and Pediatric Patients
National Board of Respiratory Care (NBRC) Testing Questions
Case Studies 1 and 2

CHAPTER OBJECTIVES

After answering the following questions, the reader should be able to:

1. Define key terms that pertain to neonatal and pediatric drug therapy
2. Explain unlabeled use of aerosolized medications
3. List and describe the most important factors affecting neonatal and pediatric aerosol drug delivery
4. Describe the clinical response of neonatal and pediatric patients to aerosolized drugs
5. Describe special circumstances related to selection of delivery devices for neonatal and pediatric patients
6. Explain the most relevant factors to select the appropriate aerosol delivery device according to age group
7. Describe the implications of compliance and cooperation on the efficiency of aerosol delivery
8. List some of the novel inhaled therapies under investigation for pediatric patients
9. Explain lung deposition of inhaled drugs in pediatric and neonatal intubated patients

KEY TERMS AND DEFINITIONS

Match the following definitions with their terms.

1. _____ A child between the ages of 1 month and 1 year
2. _____ The dose actually reaching the trachea and beyond
3. _____ The period of time between birth and the first month of life
4. _____ Refers to the period of time between 1 month and 18 years of age
5. _____ The dose released by the aerosol device
6. _____ The dose reaching the patient's mouth or artificial airway
7. _____ The dose in the delivery device
8. _____ Use of drugs with no U.S. Food and Drug Administration (FDA)–approved labeled use

a. Emitted dose
b. Infant
c. Inhaled or delivered dose
d. Lung dose
e. Neonatal
f. Nominal dose
g. Off-label
h. Pediatric

INTRODUCTION

9. In the neonatal and pediatric population, even when an optimal device is selected, what are three important factors that can reduce lung deposition?

   a. _____

   b. _____

   c. _____

10. In your own words, what is the "pediatric rule" as it relates to the FDA?

UNLABLED USE OF DRUGS IN NEONATAL AND PEDIATRIC PATIENTS

11. Is it legal for physicians to prescribe off-label use of drugs to pediatric patients?

12. The only FDA-approved lower-concentration, unit-dose albuterol sulfate treatment for asthma in children aged 2 to 12 years is _____.

13. Drug dosing with inhaled aerosols is not based on body size and blood level but on _____ _____.

14. *Fill in the following table,* indicating the differences between neonatal and adult anatomy and respiratory parameters that would affect aerosol penetration and deposition.

	Neonate	Adult
a. Tracheal length		
b. Tidal volume		
c. Minute ventilation		
d. Respiratory rate		
e. Inspiratory flow rate		

FACTORS AFFECTING NEONATAL AND PEDIATRIC AEROSOL DRUG DELIVERY

15. List three reasons that children inhale a smaller percentage of the emitted dose from either a small volume nebulizer (SVN) or metered dose inhaler (MDI) with a reservoir device.

    a. _____

    b. _____

    c. _____

16. The following is a list of factors that may affect the dose inhaled from a reservoir chamber by neonatal and pediatric patients. *Identify each as either (1) a mechanical and design factor or (2) a patient factor.*

    a. _____ Electrostatic charge on plastic devices
    b. _____ Tidal volume
    c. _____ Presence of inspiratory valve
    d. _____ Inspiratory flow rate
    e. _____ Amount of dead volume in mouthpiece

    1. Mechanical and design factor
    2. Patient factor

17. A crying infant has _____ lung deposition and _____ gastrointestinal (GI) tract deposition.

CLINICAL RESPONSE TO AEROSOLIZED DRUGS IN NEONATAL AND PEDIATRIC PATIENTS

18. Why may a younger patient (younger than 18 months of age) not have as great a clinical response to medication compared with an older child?

19. What outcome measures have documented clinical efficacy of aerosolized bronchodilators with infants?

SELECTION OF DELIVERY DEVICES

20. Name the current methods used to deliver therapeutic aerosols.

21. List the type of aerosol system that can be used for each of the age groups listed.

    a. Neonate: _____

    b. Child 5 years of age or older: _____

    c. Child 4 years of age or older: _____

    d. Child up to 4 years of age: _____

22. Although pressurized MDIs (pMDIs) may be routinely used, why may a nebulizer be a preferred method of delivery of aerosolized medication?

23. Why is a dry powder inhaler (DPI) not appropriate for children younger than 5 years?

COMPLIANCE AND COOPERATION DURING AEROSOL THERAPY

24. Applying a face mask to a child may cause crying. What are three effects produced by crying that will negatively affect aerosol delivery?

    a. _____

    b. _____

    c. _____

25. In one study, crying led to more extrathoracic aerosol deposition and greater risks of _____ _____.

26. Dose variability depends more on _____ and less on _____ design.

27. Using a "blow-by" technique reduces inhaled drug mass. Even a gap as small as 0.5 cm can reduce inhaled drug mass as much as _____ %.

28. A nebulizer _____ has shown to be more effective for aerosol delivery than is mask delivery in infants.

AEROSOL ADMINISTRATION IN INTUBATED NEONATAL AND PEDIATRIC PATIENTS

29. List three potential problems that may occur with an externally powered nebulizer placed inline on a pediatric and neonatal ventilator.

    a. _____

    b. _____

    c. _____

30. A _____/_____ nebulizer can be used inline with mechanical ventilation because it does not require external gas to power the nebulizer.

31. Most studies show a slightly higher lung deposition with the pMDI placed between the _____ piece and _____ _____.

32. Aerosol delivery may be less effective with _____ ventilation versus mechanical ventilation.

33. To improve lung deposition, the pMDI should be activated _____ _____.

NATIONAL BOARD OF RESPIRATORY CARE (NBRC) TESTING QUESTIONS

1. A person in the first 4 weeks of postnatal life is correctly termed which of the following?
   a. Postmature neonate
   b. Neonate
   c. Infant
   d. Baby

2. The lack of neonatal and pediatric _____ _____ for many drugs given by inhaled aerosol complicates aerosol delivery.
   a. Side effects
   b. Topical application
   c. Label identification
   d. Dose labeling

3. Why are SVNs not effective when treating infants with an inspiratory flow rate of less than 100 mL/sec?
   a. They would not completely inhale all of the nebulizer output during the inspiratory phase
   b. The noise is irritating to them
   c. They fall asleep before the treatment is over
   d. No research has been done to prove it works

4. Which aerosol delivery devices can be used to treat a 5-year-old patient?
   1. SVN
   2. MDI with spacer
   3. DPI
   4. Breath actuated MDI
      a. 1 and 2
      b. 2 and 3
      c. 1, 3, and 4
      d. 1, 2, 3, and 4

5. Aerosol deposition in the neonate can be affected by which of the following?
   1. Decreased inspiratory flow rate
   2. Smaller tidal volume
   3. Smaller airways
   4. Shorter respiratory cycle
      a. 1 and 2 only
      b. 2 and 3 only
      c. 1, 2, and 4 only
      d. 1, 2, 3, and 4

6. Which of the following applies to a DPI?
   a. Requires that the user generate more than 60 L/min of flow
   b. Should be used only with a spacer
   c. Can be done with an endotracheal tube
   d. All of the above

7. The dose of drug that is released from the aerosol device is called the:
   a. Inhaled dose
   b. Target dose
   c. Emitted dose
   d. Lung dose

8. Which of the following is the normal tidal volume for a neonate?
   a. 2 mL/kg
   b. 3 mL/kg
   c. 4 mL/kg
   d. 6 mL/kg

9. The only FDA-approved lower-concentration, unit-dose albuterol sulfate treatment for asthma in children aged 2 to 12 years is _____.
   a. NebuPak
   b. AccuNeb
   c. NebuLak
   d. AlbuNeb

10. You are administering an SVN aerosol to a 9-year-old asthmatic child. The amount of albuterol you place in the SVN is called the:
    a. Nominal dose
    b. Lung dose
    c. Effective dose
    d. Target dose

11. The delivered dose of medication from an SVN, MDI, or DPI that actually reaches the trachea and beyond is the _____ dose.
    a. Emitted
    b. Lung
    c. Target
    d. Specific

12. The actual dose of an inhaled aerosol drug in neonates can be as low as:
    a. Less than 1%
    b. 5%
    c. 10%
    d. 15%

13. Which of the following patient factors affect the dose inhaled from a reservoir chamber?
    1. Inspiratory flow rate
    2. Tidal volume
    3. Respiratory cycle
    4. Position of the patient in bed
        a. 1 and 3
        b. 2 and 3
        c. 1, 2, and 3
        d. 1, 2, 3, and 4

14. Administration of nebulized aerosol with a face mask using the "blow-by" technique can reduce the inhaled drug mass in a pediatric patient as much as:
    a. 50%
    b. 10%
    c. 5%
    d. 1%

15. Although pMDIs may be routinely used, a nebulizer is a preferred method of delivery of which of the following?
    a. Delivery of mucolytic agents
    b. Delivery of corticosteroids
    c. Delivery of leukotriene modifiers
    d. Delivery of hypertonic saline for cough induction

16. When using an externally powered nebulizer inline on a mechanical ventilator, which of the following are potential problems that can occur?
    1. Increased volume or pressure
    2. Bias flow interference with patient triggering
    3. Increased levels of positive end-expiratory pressure (PEEP)
    4. Variable fraction of inspired oxygen (Fio_2)
        a. 1 and 2 only
        b. 2 and 3 only
        c. 1, 2, and 4 only
        d. 1, 2, 3, and 4

17. To improve lung deposition of a patient receiving mechanical ventilation, when should the pMDI be activated?
    a. During inspiration
    b. At the end of expiration
    c. At the beginning of expiration
    d. Only during a spontaneous breath

18. Which of the following would you suggest to use to administer aerosolized medication treatment to a 2-month-old infant who is crying?
    a. Fish mask
    b. Blow-by aerosol T-piece with corrugated tubing
    c. Hood
    d. Dragon mask

19. Drug dosing with inhaled aerosols is not based on body size and blood level but based on _____ _____.
    a. Side effect
    b. GI effect
    c. Target effect
    d. Cooperation

20. What is the ideal volume for a spacer device for an infant?
    a. Small enough to allow drug inhalation with a few breaths with tidal volumes 150 to 200 mL.
    b. Small enough to allow drug inhalation with a few breaths with tidal volumes 125 to 150 mL.
    c. Small enough to allow drug inhalation with a few breaths with tidal volumes 75 to 100 mL.
    d. Small enough to allow drug inhalation with a few breaths with tidal volumes less than 50 mL.

CASE STUDY 1

A 2-month-old infant girl has been admitted to the hospital from the emergency department. The mother states her child has had a fever, persistent cough, and wheezing over the last 2 days. On assessment, the infant has a respiratory rate of 42 breaths/min, her pulse is 136 beats/min, and her temperature is 39° C. Further assessment reveals accessory muscle use and some nasal flaring. Auscultation findings include bilateral expiratory wheeze and coarse crackles in the upper lobes. The respiratory therapist suggests that the infant should receive aerosol therapy using albuterol.

1. What delivery devices are available to you?

2. Which method of delivery would you select? Justify your selection.

3. As you begin the treatment, she starts to cry and thrashes around on your lap, thus making it difficult for her to receive an effective treatment. What should you do?

4. Three days later, the child is doing much better and is being discharged. The child has been ordered to receive albuterol while at home. What delivery device should the respiratory therapist recommend for home use?

CASE STUDY 2

A 6-year-old child is in the intensive care unit and is receiving volume control mechanical ventilation. The child has the following settings:
   Mode: Assist control
   Tidal volume: 150 mL
   Rate: 20/min
   PEEP: 5 cm H_2O
   Fio_2: 0.50

Respiratory assessment reveals bilateral expiratory wheezing with coarse crackles. Over the past few hours, the pressure on the ventilator has steadily increased, indicating greater airway resistance. The respiratory therapist, according to protocol, begins administering levalbuterol every 4 hours.

1. What formulation of FDA-approved levalbuterol is available for administration to this patient receiving mechanical ventilation?

2. What is the amount of FDA-approved levalbuterol available by these formulations?

3. The respiratory therapist consults with the pulmonologists concerning the levalbuterol treatments being delivered via pMDI. The physician would like levalbuterol to be administered using an SVN. The ventilator does not have a nebulizer function to power the nebulizer, so the therapist is considering using an externally powered gas source (wall flow meter) to power the nebulizer. Are they any problems that you would want to discuss with the physician with the use of this method of nebulization?

4. The physician still wants a nebulizer to be used for the administration of albuterol. Is another option available for nebulization of medications?

5. The therapist gives this option to the doctor, and the doctor asks: "What about taking the patient off the ventilator and manually ventilating during aerosol administration?" What should be the therapist's response to this question?

6. The doctor finally agrees with your suggestion for nebulizing albuterol. Now the doctor's concern is where the nebulizer should be placed to obtain the greatest deposition of medication. What should the therapist recommend?

UNIT THREE CRITICAL CARE, CARDIOVASCULAR, AND POLYSOMNOGRAPHY AGENTS

18 Skeletal Muscle Relaxants (Neuromuscular Blocking Agents)

CHAPTER OUTLINE

Key Terms and Definitions
Uses of Neuromuscular Blocking Agents
Physiology of the Neuromuscular Junction
Nondepolarizing Agents
Depolarizing Agents
Neuromuscular Blocking Agents and Mechanical Ventilation
Monitoring of Neuromuscular Blockade
National Board of Respiratory Care (NBRC) Testing Questions
Case Studies 1 and 2

CHAPTER OBJECTIVES

After answering the following questions, the reader should be able to:

1. Define terms that pertain to skeletal muscle relaxants
2. Define neuromuscular blocking agents (NMBAs)
3. List the uses of NMBAs
4. Describe physiology of the neuromuscular junction
5. Describe the makeup of nondepolarizing agents
6. Describe the makeup of depolarizing agents
7. Describe uses of NMBAs and mechanical ventilation
8. Identify methods of monitoring neuromuscular blockade

KEY TERMS AND DEFINITIONS

Match the following definitions with their terms.

1. _____ This is the accidental inhalation of food particles, fluids, or gastric contents into the lungs

2. _____ One of the basic functional units of the nervous system that is specialized to transmit electrical nerve impulses and carry information from one part of the body to another; it consists of a cell body, axons, and dendrites

3. _____ Pneumonia that is acquired in a health care setting

4. _____ A chemical that is released from a nerve ending to transmit an impulse from a nerve cell to another nerve, muscle, organ, or other tissue

5. _____ Characteristics of a substance or drug with the ability to cause total or partial loss of memory

a. Acetylcholinesterase (AchE)
b. Amnestic properties
c. Aspiration
d. Fasciculations
e. Myasthenia gravis
f. Neuromuscular blocking agent (NMBA)
g. Neuron (nerve cell)
h. Neurotransmitter
i. Nosocomial pneumonia
j. Sedation
k. Status asthmaticus
l. Status epilepticus
m. Receptor
n. Somatic motor neurons

6. _____ Involuntary contractions or twitching of groups of muscle fibers

7. _____ An enzyme that breaks down the neurotransmitter acetylcholine at the synaptic cleft, so that the next nerve impulse can be transmitted across the synaptic gap

8. _____ The production of a restful state of mind, particularly by the use of drugs that have a calming effect, relieving anxiety and tension

9. _____ An autoimmune neuromuscular disorder characterized by chronic fatigue and exhaustion of muscles

10. _____ A person having at least 30 minutes of continuous seizure activity without full recovery between seizures

11. _____ A substance that interferes with the neural transmission between motor neurons and skeletal muscles

12. _____ An attack of asthma lasting for more than 24 hours

13. _____ A molecular structure inside or outside the cell that binds to a specific substance to elicit a physiologic response

14. _____ is part of the nervous system that controls muscles that are under voluntary control

USES OF NEUROMUSCULAR BLOCKING AGENTS

15. Explain the difference between the mechanism of action for depolarizing and nondepolarizing agents.

16. Name the only depolarizing drug currently available.

17. List eight clinical uses of NMBAs.

   a. _____
   b. _____
   c. _____
   d. _____
   e. _____
   f. _____
   g. _____
   h. _____

18. The most common pathologic condition requiring a patient to be placed on mechanical ventilation and require muscle relaxation is _____ _____.

PHYSIOLOGY OF THE NEUROMUSCULAR JUNCTION

19. The somatic motor nervous system, or skeletal muscle system, controls _____ movement.

20. The _____, which is the major muscle of ventilation, is an example of the skeletal muscle control by the somatic nervous system.

21. The autonomic nervous system controls _____ movement.

22. The transmission of nerve conduction in skeletal muscle is chemically mediated by the neurotransmitter _____.

23. Acetylcholine is then broken down and inactivated by the enzyme _____, allowing the muscle fiber to repolarize.

24. Based on neuromuscular physiology, describe two ways muscle contraction may be blocked.

    a. _____

    b. _____

NONDEPOLARIZING AGENTS

25. Nondepolarizing agents cause muscle paralysis by affecting the postsynaptic cholinergic receptors at the _____ _____.

26. _____ is an example of a cholinesterase inhibitor that can reverse nondepolarizing agents.

27. Nondepolarizing agents have a longer duration of action than the depolarizing agent _____.

28. _____ has the greatest potential to cause cardiovascular side effects, especially tachycardia and hypertension.

29. What are two concerns to respiratory therapists when administering nondepolarizing agents?

    a. _____

    b. _____

30. Which reversal agent is used to treat myasthenia gravis?

31. What drug is used to reverse succinylcholine?

32. Explain the term *Hofmann degradation* as it relates to elimination of atracurium and cistracurium.

33. What two NMBAs would not be recommended for a patient with high blood pressure and tachycardia?

    a. _____

    b. _____

34. List two side effects of reversing agents.

    a. _____

    b. _____

DEPOLARIZING AGENTS

35. List the only depolarizing agent available in the United States and its main indication for use.

36. Fill in the chart below.

Depolarizing Agent	Intravenous (IV) Dose	Time to Total Muscle Paralysis (seconds)	Clinical Duration (minutes)

37. List seven adverse effects of succinylcholine that can occur in adult patients:

   a. _____

   b. _____

   c. _____

   d. _____

   e. _____

   f. _____

   g. _____

NEUROMUSCULAR BLOCKING AGENTS AND MECHANICAL VENTILATION

38. List six disease states in which neuromuscular blockade may be beneficial.

   a. _____

   b. _____

   c. _____

   d. _____

   e. _____

   f. _____

39. In paralyzed patients receiving mechanical ventilation, elevating the head may reduce the risk of _____.

40. It is important to remember that NMBAs only cause muscle paralysis. What should be administered to remove conscious awareness and to provide pain relief?

41. _____ agents are preferred for paralysis of ventilated patients because of the predictability, longer duration of action and, manageable side effects of these agents.

MONITORING OF NEUROMUSCULAR BLOCKADE

42. List five clinical factors that can potentiate the effects of neuromuscular blockade.

   a. _____

   b. _____

   c. _____

   d. _____

   e. _____

43. List two clinical factors that can inhibit the effects of neuromuscular blockade.

    a. _____

    b. _____

44. List, in order of occurrence, the sequence of paralysis of the skeletal muscles that can be monitored physically.

    1. _____

    2. _____

    3. _____

    4. _____

    5. _____

    6. _____

    7. _____

45. During brief periods of paralysis, two simple measures of voluntary muscular function include subjective assessments such as:

    a. _____

    b. _____

46. If you were able to develop the perfect NMBA, what characteristics would it possess?

NATIONAL BOARD OF RESPIRATORY CARE (NBRC) TESTING QUESTIONS

1. Which of the following are indications for administration of an NMBA?
    1. Endotracheal extubation
    2. Muscle paralysis during surgery
    3. To facilitate mechanical ventilation
    4. Endotracheal intubation
        a. 1 and 2
        b. 3 and 4
        c. 2, 3, and 4
        d. 1, 2, 3, and 4

2. If a mechanically ventilated patient is receiving vecuronium, the patient should also receive which of the following?
    1. Sedation
    2. Analgesics
    3. Frequent suctioning
    4. Bronchodilator therapy
        a. 1 and 2 only
        b. 1 and 3 only
        c. 2, 3, and 4 only
        d. 1, 2, 3, and 4

3. Which of the following best defines an NMBA?
    a. Drugs that partially block selected skeletal muscles, such as the diaphragm
    b. Drugs that reduce heart rate and blood pressure during invasive medical procedures
    c. Drugs that minimize brain activity for traumatic brain injury
    d. Drugs that paralyze muscles and prevent movement

4. Which of the following is currently the only depolarizing NMBA?
   a. Atracurium
   b. Cisatracurium
   c. Pancuronium
   d. Succinylcholine

5. Muscle paralysis caused by nondepolarizing blocking agents can be reversed using which of the following?
   a. Cholinesterase
   b. Cholinesterase inhibitors
   c. Parasympatholytics
   d. Sympathomimetics

6. The transmission of nerve conduction in skeletal muscle is chemically mediated by which neurotransmitter?
   a. Acetylcholine
   b. Serotonin
   c. Acetylcholinesterase
   d. Norepinephrine

7. Which of the following drugs can reverse the effects of nondepolarizing blockade?
   1. Edrophonium
   2. Pyridostigmine
   3. Neostigmine
   4. Rocuronium
      a. 1 and 2 only
      b. 1, 2, and 3 only
      c. 2, 3, and 4 only
      d. 1, 2, 3, and 4

8. A cardiac patient requires intubation and mechanical ventilation. Which of the following NMBAs should be administered to minimize any potential for cardiac side effects?
   a. Vecuronium
   b. Atropine
   c. Pancuronium
   d. Succinylcholine

9. The neuromuscular drug of choice to assist in endotracheal intubation is:
   a. Vecuronium
   b. Atracurium
   c. Mivacurium
   d. Succinylcholine

10. For endotracheally intubated, paralyzed patients receiving mechanical ventilation, which of the following may help reduce the risk of aspiration?
    a. Reduce the ventilator driving pressure
    b. Elevate the head of the bed
    c. Have the patient supine with legs raised
    d. Reduce the positive end-expiratory pressure (PEEP) to less than 5 cm H_2O.

11. What is the intravenous dose for succinylcholine?
    a. 0.3-1.0 mg/kg
    b. 0.5-0.8 mg/kg
    c. 1.0-1.5 mg/kg
    d. 2.0-2.5 mg/kg

12. What is the simplest means of monitoring the adequacy of neuromuscular blockade?
    a. Train of four
    b. Twitch monitoring
    c. Response to painful stimuli
    d. Direct observation of muscle activity

13. What would likely be the first indication that a nondepolarizing agent is reversing?
    a. Eyelids move, and the eyes move back and forth
    b. Extremities move with twitching and spasms
    c. The diaphragm contracts indicated by abdominal wall movement
    d. The patient swallows and coughs

14. During brief periods of paralysis, which of the following subjective assessments measures voluntary muscular functions?
    1. Hand grip strength
    2. The ability to lift the head off the bed for 5 seconds
    3. Heart rate returning to normal
    4. Increase in SpO_2
        a. 1 and 2 only
        b. 2 and 3 only
        c. 1, 3, and 4 only
        d. 1, 2, and 4 only

15. Repolarization of the muscle fiber occurs when acetylcholine is broken down and inactivated by the enzyme:
    a. Acetylcholinesterase
    b. Neostigmine
    c. Cholinesterase
    d. Acetylcholine

16. Nondepolarizing agents cause muscle paralysis by affecting the postsynaptic cholinergic receptors at the:
    a. Synaptic cleft
    b. Neuromuscular junction
    c. Dendrite
    d. Neuroeffector site

17. When a nondepolarizing agent is administered in a nonintubated patient, what should the respiratory therapist be concerned with?
    1. The intracranial pressures
    2. Maintaining a patent airway
    3. The appropriate size suction catheter to be used
    4. Maintaining appropriate ventilation
        a. 2 and 4
        b. 1 and 3
        c. 1, 2, and 4
        d. 1, 2, 3, and 4

18. To reduce the adverse effects of NMBAs, which of the following medications can be given?
    a. Atropine
    b. Neostigmine
    c. Edrophonium
    d. Quafenisine

19. Which of the following indicates initial depolarization after administration of succinylcholine?
    a. Tachycardia
    b. Hypertension
    c. Fasciculations
    d. Paralysis

20. Which of the following NMBAs cannot be reversed with medication?
    a. Pancuronium
    b. Succinylcholine
    c. Rocuronium
    d. Vecuronium

CASE STUDY 1

You are called to the emergency department to assist in the care of patient who was in a motor vehicle accident. In the report, you learn that he has pulmonary contusions and a flail chest. He is not responding to verbal commands and is combative. On the basis of his arterial blood gases and other physical findings, you recommend that the patient be orally intubated.

1. Which NMBA would you use to paralyze him? Why?

The patient is intubated and moved to the intensive care unit, where he is placed on mechanical ventilation. Over the next few hours, the patient remains very restless. He is breathing asynchronously with the ventilator in spite of several changes made to the ventilator settings. Physical assessment reveals:
   Respiratory rate: 30 breaths/min
   Blood pressure: 170/100 mm Hg
   Pulse: 148 beats/min
   You call the physician and suggest an NMBA.

2. Which classification of NMBA would you recommend?

3. Based on the patient's physical assessment, what agents would be most appropriate to use? Why?

4. What type of blocking agent would you *not* want to use for this patient, and why?

5. Are there any other medications you would suggest for this patient receiving NMBAs?

The patient has been given an NMBA, is now paralyzed, and has received a sedative and pain medication.

6. How could you determine that the patient received an appropriate amount of medication to reduce pain and anxiety adequately?

7. Because clinical signs are lost with paralysis, what should be monitored continuously to assess signs of restlessness, anxiety, and distress?

CASE STUDY 2

A patient diagnosed with severe asthma exacerbation has been intubated and is receiving pressure-controlled ventilation. Despite numerous changes to the ventilator settings, the patient is agitated and is "fighting the ventilator," according to the respiratory therapist. The respiratory therapist has decided to call the pulmonologist for an order for an NMBA.

1. What would be a clinical indication for administration of an NMBA for this patient?

2. Which classification of NMBAs would you suggest for this patient?

3. If the physician were to ask for your recommendation about an NMBA for this patient, what agent would be least appropriate to administer? What would be the best agent to administer?

The patient is now paralyzed and is breathing synchronously with the ventilator.

4. While the patient is intubated and receiving mechanical ventilation, what can you do to reduce the incidence of nosocomial infection and aspiration while the patient is receiving an NMBA?

The next day it is decided to begin reversing the NMBA.

5. What would be a quick, subjective assessment to determine the depth of blockade and voluntary muscle function?

6. What could you use to assess the patient's muscle strength objectively?

The physician has now administered a reversing agent.

7. What would be the first response indicating the patient has begun breathing on his own?

19 Diuretic Agents

CHAPTER OUTLINE

Key Terms and Definitions
Renal Structure and Function
Diuretic Groups
Diuretics and Acute Respiratory Distress Syndrome
National Board of Respiratory Care (NBRC) Testing Questions
Case Studies 1 and 2

CHAPTER OBJECTIVES

After answering the following questions, the reader should be able to:

1. Define terms pertaining to diuretic agents
2. Describe renal function, filtration, reabsorption, and acid-base balance
3. List and describe the various groups of diuretics
4. List some of the indications for diuretic therapy
5. List the most common adverse reactions associated with the use of diuretics
6. Describe special situations related to diuretic therapy

KEY TERMS AND DEFINITIONS

Match the following definitions with their terms.

1. _____ Swelling resulting from an abnormal accumulation of fluid in intercellular spaces of the body

2. _____ Abnormally decreased volume of blood circulating in the body

3. _____ The microscopic functional unit of the kidney responsible for filtering and maintaining fluid balance; each kidney is made of approximately 2 million of these

4. _____ Inadequacy of the heart as a pump, failing to maintain adequacy of blood circulation, with resulting congestion and tissue edema

5. _____ Amount of urine produced in 24 hours; normal urine output averages 30-60 mL/hour

6. _____ The return to the blood of most of the water, sodium (Na^+), amino acids, and sugar that were removed during filtration; occurs mainly in the proximal tubule of the nephron

7. _____ The mechanism by which the hydrostatic pressure forces fluid out of the glomerular capillary into the renal ducts

a. Congestive heart failure (CHF)
b. Edema
c. Glomerular filtration
d. Hypovolemia
e. Nephrocalcinosis
f. Nephron
g. Ototoxicity
h. Reabsorption
i. Synergistic effect
j. Urine output
k. Diuretic

8. _____ Renal lithiasis in which calcium deposits form in the renal parenchyma and result in reduced kidney function and the presence of blood in the urine

9. _____ Damage to the ear, specifically the cochlea or auditory nerve and sometimes the vestibulum, by a toxin

10. _____ Situation in which the effect of two chemicals on an organism is greater than the effect of each chemical individually

11. _____ A drug that increases urine output

RENAL STRUCTURE AND FUNCTION

12. List the three basic functions of the renal system.

    a. _____

    b. _____

    c. _____

13. From which artery does the kidney receive blood flow?

Review Box 19-1 in the textbook for ions that are filtered and exchanged in the kidneys.

14. What is the name of the hormone produced by the posterior pituitary gland that aids in the regulation of urine output?

15. From where is aldosterone secreted?

16. Explain how an increase in a patient's preload can result in an increased urine output.

17. _____ or _____ will force Na^+ exchange for H^+, thereby producing metabolic alkalosis.

18. Most filtered K^+ is reabsorbed in the proximal tubules. The K^+ found in the urine is that secreted by the _____.

19. Chloride and bicarbonate are passively reabsorbed in the _____ and _____.

DIURETIC GROUPS

20. What is the main purpose of diuretics?

21. How do most diuretics work?

22. One of the most common uses of osmotic diuretics is for the treatment of _____ _____.

23. Osmotic substances are potent diuretics that lead to increased excretion of _____ and _____.

24. List three common uses for carbonic anhydrase inhibitors (CAIs).

    a. _____

    b. _____

    c. _____

25. Explain the mechanism of action for loop diuretics.

26. Loop diuretics are administered to patients with pulmonary edema to cause _____.

27. Apart from their diuretic effects, loop diuretics may cause an acute _____ effect.

28. How long after administration of a loop diuretic should diuresis take place? What would you suggest to the physician if it does not happen?

29. What is the mechanism of action for thiazide diuretics? Why are they not as potent as other diuretics?

30. List a clinical indication for the administration of thiazide diuretics.

31. Explain the mechanism of action for K⁺-sparing diuretics.

32. The most common diuretic combination is _____ and _____.

33. List three major complications or adverse effects of diuretics.

    a. _____

    b. _____

    c. _____

34. List three indications for K⁺ supplementation.

    a. _____

    b. _____

    c. _____

35. An increased blood glucose level, referred to as _____, is associated with the use of loop and thiazide diuretics.

36. One of the least toxic and most effective loop diuretics in pediatric practice is _____.

DIURETICS AND ACUTE RESPIRATORY DISTRESS SYNDROME

37. According to the Fluid and Catheter Treatment Trial (FACTT), what three positive outcomes were the result of conservative fluid management for acute respiratory distress syndrome (ARDS)?

    a. _____

    b. _____

    c. _____

NATIONAL BOARD OF RESPIRATORY CARE (NBRC) TESTING QUESTIONS

1. Urine output less than 30 to 60 mL/hour is known as _____.
   a. Polyuria
   b. Anuria
   c. Oliguria
   d. Nephronemia

2. Carbonic anhydrase inhibitors act in which of the following?
   a. Proximal tubules
   b. Distal tubules
   c. Loop of Henle
   d. Glomerulus

3. Approximately what percentage of the cardiac output in a normal 70-kg adult flows through the kidneys?
   a. 10
   b. 15
   c. 20
   d. 22

4. Potassium-sparing diuretics interfere with the sodium/potassium exchange in the:
   a. Distal convulated tubule
   b. Loop of Henle
   c. Proximal tubule
   d. Bladder

5. Normal urine output averages:
   a. 10 to 30 mL/hour
   b. 30 to 60 mL/hour
   c. 100 to 120 mL/hour
   d. 120 to 140 mL/hour

6. Which of the following is the most common combination of diuretics?
   a. Mannitol and thiazide
   b. Loop and carbonic anhydrase inhibitor
   c. Thiazide and carbonic anhydrase inhibitor
   d. Loop and thiazide

7. The functional unit of the kidneys is called the:
   a. Ureter
   b. Nephron
   c. Urethra
   d. Loop of Henle

8. The K^+ found in the urine is that secreted by which of the following?
   a. Distal tubule
   b. Proximal tubule
   c. Nephrons
   d. Central tubules

9. Osmotic diuretics are potent diuretics that lead to increased excretion of which of the following?
   a. Magnesium
   b. Glucose and water
   c. Water and NaCl
   d. Sodium

10. If a patient has hypokalemia, which of the following acid-base disturbances is most likely?
    a. Respiratory acidosis
    b. Metabolic alkalosis
    c. Respiratory alkalosis
    d. Metabolic acidosis

11. The drug of choice to treat cerebral edema is:
    a. Furosemide
    b. Diamox
    c. Mannitol
    d. Benzthiazide

12. Patients receiving loop diuretics should have _____ levels monitored.
    a. Bicarbonate
    b. pH
    c. Bleeding time
    d. Electrolytes

13. A patient receiving loop diuretics should experience diuresis within:
    a. 1 hour
    b. 20 minutes
    c. 2 hours
    d. 24 hours

14. The main reason for administering a loop diuretic to a patient with pulmonary edema is:
    a. To reduce inflammation in the airways
    b. To cause pulmonary artery vasoconstriction and reduce pulmonary vascular resistance
    c. To increase left heart pressure
    d. To cause diuresis and reduce pulmonary edema

15. For pediatric patients, the least toxic and most effective diuretic is:
    a. Mannitol
    b. CAI
    c. Furosemide
    d. Isosorbide

16. Within 5 minutes of the administration of intravenous loop diuretics to cardiac patients, which of the following effects is observed?
    a. Vasoconstriction
    b. Vasodilation
    c. Edema
    d. Hypertonicity

17. Osmotic diuretics are often used in the management of which of the following?
    a. Traumatic brain injury
    b. Kidney failure
    c. Ascites
    d. Liver failure

18. Thiazide diuretics are considered to be first line of therapy for which of the following?
    a. Left heart failure
    b. Cor pulmonale
    c. Mild hypertension
    d. Acute renal failure

19. Which of the following are the most common side effects of diuretic therapy?
    1. Hypervolemia
    2. Hypovolemia
    3. Reduced cerebral perfusion
    4. Acid-base abnormalities
       a. 1 and 3
       b. 2 and 4
       c. 2, 3, and 4
       d. 1, 3, and 4

20. Although CAIs are considered to be very weak diuretics, they are commonly used to treat which of the following?
    1. Glaucoma
    2. Metabolic alkalosis
    3. Motion sickness
    4. Altitude sickness
       a. 1 and 2
       b. 1, 2, and 3
       c. 2, 3, and 4
       d. 1, 2, and 4

CASE STUDY 1

Mrs. S. has been brought to the emergency department (ED) with chief complaints of increasing shortness of breath, coughing, and mild substernal pressure. Her husband called the paramedics when she complained she "cannot breathe." Mrs. S. is currently on a Venturi mask with an inspired oxygen fraction (Fio_2) of 0.50. Her husband states she is a 66-year-old housewife with a history of coronary artery disease, arrhythmia, and a recent hospitalization for 3 weeks, resulting from an anterior wall myocardial infarction (MI); she has been out of the hospital for a month. Physical examination reveals a heart rate of 158 beats/min, blood pressure of 110/70 mm Hg, and a Spo_2 of 93% on the Venturi mask. Breath sounds reveal inspiratory crackles from the bases up to the midchest, with mild expiratory wheezes. Her respiratory rate is 34 breaths/min, with some paradoxical respirations noted. Pitting edema is present in the ankles, no clubbing or cyanosis is noted, and her skin is cool and diaphoretic. There is jugular vein distention noted.

Mrs. S. has been admitted to the cardiac care unit. A portable chest radiograph taken on admission in the ED has now been returned and reveals cardiomegaly, as well as bilateral pulmonary vascular engorgement with interstitial and alveolar edema. She is diagnosed with congestive heart failure.

1. What drug would be beneficial in helping to remove fluid from the patient's lungs?

2. Thirty minutes after giving 40 mg of Lasix, diuresis has not occurred. What would you now recommend?

It has been 2 hours since Mrs. S. was admitted to the cardiac care unit. She is resting more comfortably and is on a nasal cannula at 3 L/minute. Because of the medications she is currently receiving, laboratory tests are obtained with the following results:
   Potassium: 2.5 mEq/L (normal: 3.5-5.0 mEq/L)
   Sodium: 140 mEq/L (normal: 136-145 mEq/L)
   Chloride: 87 mEq/L (normal: 95-105 mEq/L)
   Glucose: 125 mg/dL (normal: 90-150 mg/dL)

3. On the basis of this finding, what would you recommend?

4. What acid-base imbalance is likely to occur with these chemistry results?

CASE STUDY 2

You are the day shift supervisor for a 300-bed hospital in the respiratory therapy department. You are making rounds in the morning when your beeper alerts you to come to the ED.

A patient has been admitted with severe headache. Blood pressure is 160/100 mm Hg, pulse is 128 beats/min, and respirations are 26 breaths/min. Chest radiograph reveals a normal size heart, and the lungs are normal. After administering oxygen to the patient, it has been decided to administer a diuretic.

1. Which diuretic class would best for this patient?

2. Explain the action of this diuretic.

You are now called to the intensive care unit, where a patient has been admitted after a motorcycle accident. The patient has sustained a head injury. Computed tomography scan shows contusions and brain swelling. The patient has been placed on mechanical ventilation.

3. Which diuretic class would be indicated for this patient?

4. Explain the action of this diuretic.

This patient has now been stabilized, and you are paged to the ED. On entering the ED, you are informed that a 75-year-old man has complaints of severe eye pain, nausea, and vomiting. The patient's eyes are red, and he complains of blurred vision.

5. What diuretic class would be most helpful for this patient's condition?

6. Explain the action of this diuretic.

20 Drugs Affecting the Central Nervous System

CHAPTER OUTLINE

Key Terms and Definitions
Brain Structure and Function
Neurotransmitters
Psychiatric Medications
    Antidepressants
    Mood Stabilizers
    Antipsychotics
    Drugs for Alzheimer's Dementia: Cholinesterase Inhibitors
    Anxiolytics
    Barbiturates and Other Hypnotics
Ethyl Alcohol
Pain Treatment
    Conscious Sedation
Central Nervous System and Respiratory Stimulants
National Board of Respiratory Care (NBRC) Testing Questions
Case Studies 1 and 2

CHAPTER OBJECTIVES

After answering the following questions, the reader should be able to:

1. Define key terms pertaining to drugs that affect the central nervous system
2. Describe the multiple functions of the central nervous system
3. Recognize various effects of medications on the central nervous system and their ability to modulate neurotransmitters
4. Comprehend psychiatric medications, including their classification, use, and side effect profiles
5. Recognize the effects of alcohol on the central nervous system during acute intoxication and chronic use and after abrupt withdrawal
6. Distinguish physiologic and psychological bases of pain and the classes of analgesics used to treat them
7. Recognize the indications for use of both local and general anesthesia
8. Describe the concept of conscious sedation and its indications and guidelines for use
9. Distinguish drugs that stimulate the central nervous and respiratory systems and describe the indications for application

KEY TERMS AND DEFINITIONS

Match the following definitions with their terms.

1. _____ The brain and spinal cord make up the functional components of this system; together these provide for all conscious and subconscious functions of the body

2. _____ These drugs can alter levels of certain neurotransmitters, in particular norepinephrine and serotonin within the brain

a. Analgesics
b. Anesthetics
c. Antidepressants
d. Antipsychotics
e. Anxiolytics
f. Central nervous system (CNS)
g. Cholinesterase inhibitors

3. _____ These drugs depress the nervous system; they can be divided into two categories, local and general. Their use results in the absence of pain perception

4. _____ These drugs are used primarily to treat bipolar disorders

5. _____ These drugs provide pain relief; they can be subdivided into narcotic and nonnarcotic medications

6. _____ These drugs are used to treat psychotic disorders, such as schizophrenia, and they affect primarily the neurotransmitter dopamine

7. _____ This is a method used during certain invasive procedures; the goals of this method are to decrease the level of consciousness and relieve anxiety and pain, while allowing the patient to follow verbal commands

8. _____ These drugs can cause increased activity of the brain

9. _____ These drugs are known as minor tranquilizers; they treat several conditions, including anxiety disorders and insomnia

10. _____ These drugs block the activity of cholinesterase, an enzyme that inactivates the neurotransmitter acetylcholine

11. _____ This is a chemical substance that allows neurons to transmit electrical impulses throughout the CNS and peripheral nervous system

h. Conscious sedation
i. Mood stabilizers
j. Neurotransmitter
k. Stimulants

BRAIN STRUCTURE AND FUNCTION

12. Give a brief description of the following areas of the brain.
    a. Cortex
    b. Midbrain
    c. Brainstem or medulla

13. What disease is caused by a loss of neurons containing dopamine in the midbrain and is characterized by resting tremor and gait disturbances?

NEUROTRANSMITTERS

14. The clinical effects of CNS drugs depend on what factor?

15. Do CNS drugs increase or decrease individual neuronal activity?

16. The effect of the neurotransmitter released is determined by what six factors?

   a. _____

   b. _____

   c. _____

   d. _____

   e. _____

   f. _____

PSYCHIATRIC MEDICATIONS

Antidepressants

17. Deficiency of what two neurotransmitters has been linked to depression?

18. List three etiologies of depressive disorders.

   a. _____

   b. _____

   c. _____

19. Fill in the U.S. brand names for the following drugs used to treat depression.

GENERIC DRUG	U.S. BRAND NAME
Citalopram	
Fluoxetine	
Paroxetine	
Duloxetine	
Bupropion	
Mirtazapine	
Phenelzine	

Mood Stabilizers

20. Pharmacologic treatment of bipolar disorder typically begins with a _____ _____.

21. _____ disorder involves alternating episodes of depression and mania or hypomania.

Antipsychotics

22. What neurotransmitter does pharmacotherapy for psychosis associated with depression or mania generally aim to increase?

Drugs for Alzheimer's Dementia: Cholinesterase Inhibitors

23. Deficits of which neurotransmitter are associated with cognitive deficits in patients with Alzheimer's dementia?

24. What type of drug can improve cognition and function in patients with Alzheimer's disease?

Anxiolytics

25. Circle the drugs that are used to treat anxiety and insomnia.
    a. Xanax
    b. Valium
    c. Restoril
    d. Ativan
    e. Seconal

26. When given with opioids, what side effect could benzodiazepines augment?

Barbiturates and Other Hypnotics

27. When choosing a sedative drug for your patient, why would you choose a benzodiazepine over a barbiturate?

28. For the following drugs, give an indication for each of them.
    a. Thiopental: _____
    b. Pentobarbital: _____
    c. Phenobarbital: _____

29. A common complaint that frequently results in the prescription of a hypnotic is _____.

ETHYL ALCOHOL

30. What is considered a toxic level of blood alcohol? What side effect from toxic levels would concern you?

31. Abrupt withdrawal after prolonged use may result in the syndrome of _____, characterized by CNS hyperactivity, including hyperthermia, increased blood pressure, muscle twitching, hallucinosis, and seizures.

32. True or False: Alcohol is metabolized to carbon dioxide (CO_2) and water (H_2O) and produces acetaldehyde in the process.

PAIN TREATMENT

33. What is pain?

34. What are two components of the pain experience?

    a. _____

    b. _____

35. How do nonsteroidal antiinflammatory drugs (NSAIDs) work?

36. The most frequently used analgesic, an NSAID that is purchased over the counter, is _____.

37. Your patient was just brought into the emergency department (ED) in respiratory arrest after taking hydromorphone while his Duragesic patch was on. What medication would you give to reverse his respiratory depression?

38. List a reason for allowing patients to use a patient-controlled analgesia (PCA) device to control their pain.

39. Depth of anesthesia is determined by the patient's response to painful stimuli and is often judged by the sympathetic response, such as a change in _____ _____ or _____.

Conscious Sedation

40. During conscious sedation, patients should remain _____ and able to communicate, protect their own _____, and breathe adequately.

41. How many qualified people must be continuously present during the sedation period?

42. Because of the potential for airway compromise, what should the respiratory therapist have available to maintain a patent airway?

43. What recommendations for monitoring are suggested during conscious sedation?

    a. _____

    b. _____

    c. _____

    d. _____

CENTRAL NERVOUS SYSTEM AND RESPIRATORY STIMULANTS

44. _____ is a common component in popular beverages and is used therapeutically in apnea-bradycardia syndromes of premature births.

NATIONAL BOARD OF RESPIRATORY CARE (NBRC) TESTING QUESTIONS

1. The area of the brain that controls motor function and coordinates movement is the:
   a. Cerebrum
   b. Diencephalon
   c. Brainstem
   d. Cerebellum

2. Control of breathing is regulated mainly in the:
   a. Cerebrum
   b. Diencephalon
   c. Brainstem
   d. Cerebellum

3. Psychotic disorders are characterized by:
   a. Unstable gait
   b. Rigidity and hypertonicity
   c. Excessive fidgeting
   d. Impaired reality testing

4. Which of the following is considered to be a toxic level of alcohol?
   a. 200 to 300 mg/dL
   b. 325 to 400 mg/dL
   c. 425 to 500 mg/dL
   d. 400 to 600 mg/dL

5. Which class of analgesics may enhance bronchodilation and suppress cough when administered by inhalation?
   a. Alcohol
   b. NSAIDs
   c. Local anesthetics
   d. Barbiturates

6. A disease characterized by resting tremor, rigidity, and postural instability resulting from loss of dopamine-containing neurons is:
   a. Parkinson's disease
   b. Delirium tremens
   c. Manic depression
   d. Bipolar disorder

7. These drugs, subdivided into narcotic and nonnarcotic medications, provide pain relief:
   a. Anxiolytics
   b. Mood stabilizers
   c. Analgesics
   d. Cholinesterase inhibitors

8. The brain is composed of which of the following?
   1. Cortex
   2. Spinal cord
   3. Brainstem
   4. Midbrain
      a. 1 and 2
      b. 1, 3, and 4
      c. 2, 3, and 4
      d. 1, 2, 3, and 4

9. Medical treatment of any degree of bipolar disorder must begin with which of the following medications?
   a. Opioid analgesic
   b. Mood stabilizer
   c. Barbiturates
   d. Antidepressants

10. A person diagnosed with Alzheimer's disease would have improvement of cognition and function with the use of this class of drugs:
    a. Mood stabilizers
    b. Sympathomimetics
    c. Cholinesterase inhibitors
    d. Pain relievers

11. Which of the following drugs is recommended to control seizures?
    a. Thiopental
    b. Pentobarbital
    c. Norepinephrine
    d. Phenobarbital

12. As alcohol is broken down and metabolized into CO_2 and H_2O, the byproduct is:
    a. Acetaldehyde
    b. Dopamine
    c. Norepinephrine
    d. Acetylcysteine

13. Chronic pain can be controlled by antidepressants and _____.
    a. Mood stabilizers
    b. Analgesics
    c. Tranquilizers
    d. Anesthetics

14. The most frequently used analgesic NSAID that can be purchased over the counter is:
    a. Lithium
    b. Ethanol
    c. Aspirin
    d. Phenobarbital

15. Depth of anesthesia is determined by the patient's response to painful stimuli and is often judged by the sympathetic response, which is:
    a. Twitching of the extremities
    b. Lack of feeling in the extremities
    c. A change in heart rate or blood pressure
    d. A drop in arterial oxygen saturation

16. Which of the following procedures has guidelines requiring that at least the operator and a monitoring assistant must be present during administration?
    a. General anesthesia
    b. Conscious sedation
    c. Intravenous opioids
    d. Local anesthesia

17. Respiratory failure resulting from sedative or opioid drug overdose can be treated with which of the following specific antagonists?
    a. Methylxanthines
    b. Morphine
    c. Naloxone
    d. Caffeine

18. A hospitalized patient is complaining of insomnia and anxiety related to upcoming procedures. A drug that would help treat these conditions would be which of the following?
    a. Haldol
    b. Lithium
    c. Xanax
    d. Prozac

19. What is considered to be the fifth vital sign?
    a. Oxygen saturation
    b. Pain
    c. Eye movement
    d. Finger movement

20. A patient has continual complaints of pain. When asked how intense the pain is, the patient keeps saying: "It hurts." Which of the following would be a way to have the patient estimate the magnitude of the pain?
    a. Have the patient point to the painful area.
    b. Have the patient describe in detail the pain.
    c. Have the patient relate a past painful experience to this one.
    d. Use a numeric analog pain scale.

CASE STUDY 1

You are the day-shift respiratory therapy supervisor, and you will be involved in treating various patients throughout the day. Your responsibilities today will take you to the ED, the intensive care unit (ICU), labor and delivery, and the neonatal ICU. Your task, if you decide to take it, will be to assist in decision-making opportunities in treating these patients. Good luck.

You are called to the ED, where you find Mr. Jones, a 67-year-old patient with chronic obstructive pulmonary disease (COPD) who has been admitted with pneumonia. His respiratory rate is 34 breaths/min, he has prolonged exhalation and accessory muscle usage, and he is breathing with a 2-L/min nasal cannula. His arterial blood gas (ABG) shows the following: pH, 7.21; partial pressure of arterial carbon dioxide ($Paco_2$), 74 mm Hg; partial pressure of arterial oxygen (Pao_2), 49 mm Hg; bicarbonate (HCO_3), 34 mEq/L. The resident wants to give a respiratory stimulant, an analeptic drug, to stimulate his breathing to "blow off" the CO_2. You enter the patient's room just as the resident is asking the nurse to give the drug.

1. What would you recommend?

You are now called by a nurse on the floors. The nurse tells you that a patient is about to go home, and this patient would like her respiratory treatment before she leaves. After the treatment, the patient asks what you would recommend for a medication to help with her pain. She explains that the pain is getting better, but she still has mild pain and she does not want a prescription.

2. What medication would you suggest?

After leaving this patient, you are paged to labor and delivery, where a 32-week gestational age infant is born via cesarean section. The mother received several drugs, one of which was an opioid. The infant is not responding to typical stimuli and is currently being hand ventilated with a resuscitation bag.

3. What drug should be given to reverse the effects of the opioid?

From here you are called to neonatal ICU. The respiratory therapist is about to implement continuous positive airway pressure (CPAP) therapy on a 27-week infant who had been receiving mechanical ventilation. The therapist has reported to you that the infant has had some episodes of apnea, and the therapist is concerned about placing the infant on CPAP. The therapist asks you to recommend a drug that would stimulate the infant's breathing.

4. What would you recommend?

CASE STUDY 2

A patient in the ICU is about to have a medical procedure performed at the bedside. After the patient has signed the consent form, she asks what comfort measures will be administered during the procedure. You tell her that she will be receiving conscious sedation. She does not understand what this means.

1. How would you explain what conscious sedation is and how it will make her more comfortable during the procedure?

2. In preparation for the procedure, what should the respiratory therapist have available to maintain the patient's airway?

3. The patient would like to know who else will be in the room besides the respiratory therapist and how will she be monitored. What would you tell this patient?

4. As you are preparing the resuscitation equipment, the patient's nurse tells you that she has never assisted in conscious sedation. She would like to know how many people need to be present during the sedation period. What would you tell the nurse?

21 Vasopressors, Inotropes, and Antiarrhythmic Agents

CHAPTER OUTLINE

Key Terms and Definitions
Overview of the Cardiovascular System and Factors Affecting Blood Pressure
Agents Used in the Management of Shock
    Catecholamines
    Inotropic Agents
    Phosphodiesterase Inhibitors
    Cardiac Glycosides
Electrophysiology of the Myocardium
Pharmacology of Antiarrhythmics
Management and Pharmacotherapy of Advanced Cardiac Life Support
National Board of Respiratory Care (NBRC) Testing Questions
Case Studies 1 and 2

CHAPTER OBJECTIVES

After answering the following questions, the reader should be able to:

1. Define terms that pertain to vasopressors, inotropes, and antiarrhythmic drugs
2. List the various components that make up blood pressure
3. Compare and contrast the mechanism of action of inotropes and vasopressors
4. Describe the various drug interactions that may occur with the use of vasopressors and inotropes
5. Design an algorithm for the management of hypotension
6. Manage extravasation injuries that occur with use of vasopressor therapy
7. Describe the normal conduction of the heart
8. Define nonpharmacologic methods of treating dysrhythmias
9. Define the mechanism of action of digoxin
10. List all the dysrhythmias associated with cardiac arrest
11. Design an algorithm that may be used in the management of ventricular fibrillation and pulseless ventricular tachycardia
12. Design an algorithm that may be used in the management of torsades de pointes
13. Describe the proper dosing technique of intravenous (IV) magnesium therapy in the management of torsades de pointes
14. List the routes of administering medications during cardiac arrest

KEY TERMS AND DEFINITIONS

Match the following definitions with their terms.

1. _____ The presence of carbon dioxide aiding in the release and delivery of oxygen from hemoglobin

2. _____ Amount of blood that is pumped out of the heart per unit of time

3. _____ The lowest pressure reached right before ventricular ejection

a. Antiarrhythmics
b. Atrioventricular (AV) node
c. Bohr effect
d. Cardiac output (CO)
e. Catecholamines
f. Diastolic blood pressure (DBP)
g. Mean arterial pressure (MAP)
h. Phosphodiesterase

4. _____ Pressure that drives blood into the tissues, averaged over the entire cardiac cycle

5. _____ Cardiac medications that are classified according to their mechanism of action; in some instances, they may present multiple mechanisms of action

6. _____ Endogenous products that are secreted into the bloodstream and travel to nerve endings to stimulate an excitatory response

7. _____ Link between atrial depolarization and ventricular depolarization

8. _____ Peak pressure reached during ventricular ejection

9. _____ An episode of ventricular fibrillation, pulseless ventricular tachycardia, pulseless electrical activity, or asystole leading to loss of life

10. _____ An enzyme responsible for the breakdown of cyclic adenosine 3′,5′-monophosphate (cAMP)

11. _____ Irregular heartbeat

12. _____ An agent that influences the conduction of electrical impulses

13. _____ An agent affecting the rate of contraction of the heart

14. _____ A slow heart rate, typically defined as less than 60 beats/min

15. _____ An overly rapid heartbeat, usually defined as greater than 100 beats/min in adults

16. _____ A cardiac arrhythmia in which normal atrial contractions are replaced by rapid irregular twitchings of the muscular wall

17. _____ A cardiac arrhythmia in which normal ventricular contractions are replaced by rapid movements of the ventricular muscle

18. _____ Agent causing contraction of the capillaries and arteries

19. _____ An agent affecting the strength of muscular contraction

20. _____ An agent causing dilation of blood vessels

i. Sudden cardiac death (SCD)
j. Systolic blood pressure (SBP)
k. Arrhythmia/dysrhythmia
l. Chronotropic
m. Tachycardia
n. Ventricular fibrillation
o. Inotropic
p. Vasodilator
q. Vasopressor
r. Atrial fibrillation
s. Bradycardia
t. Dromotropic

OVERVIEW OF THE CARDIOVASCULAR SYSTEM AND FACTORS AFFECTING BLOOD PRESSURE

21. Tissue perfusion depends on what three factors?

    a. _____

    b. _____

    c. _____

22. If your patient was in cardiogenic shock and had a decreased cardiac output, would a pulse oximeter attached to his or her index finger be an accurate way to measure oxygenation status?

23. What is the major determinant of (a) blood pressure and (b) ventricular contractility?

24. Calculate the CO of a patient with a blood pressure of 120/70 mm Hg, a stroke volume of 70 mL/beat, and a heart rate of 80 beats/min.

25. What are two determinants of MAP?

    a. _____

    b. _____

26. Calculate the MAP of a patient who has a blood pressure of 120/90 mm Hg.

27. Define stroke volume.

List the normal pressures of each hemodynamic parameter.

28. Central venous pressure (CVP): _____

29. Pulmonary capillary wedge pressure (PCWP): _____

30. Cardiac output (CO): _____

31. Systemic vascular resistance (SVR): _____

AGENTS USED IN THE MANAGEMENT OF SHOCK

32. Your patient has just suffered severe blood loss due to the arterial line's becoming dislodged. What would be your first-line therapy to improve the hypotension?

33. Your patient's hemodynamic parameters are currently being measured. If the patient were fluid overloaded, what measurement would likely be altered? Would it increase or decrease?

34. List a clinical indication for the use of Levophed.

Catecholamines

35. After administration of epinephrine, stimulation of what receptor type is likely to produce a net effect of tachycardia?

36. Isoproterenol can be used to relax the smooth muscle of the bronchi. Why is its use limited? What is its brand name?

37. The medical student suggests the use of dopamine to treat a patient in septic shock. You suggest norepinephrine. How would you explain your choice and why it is the more appropriate pharmacologic treatment for the patient to the attending physician?

38. Explain why your patient receiving a phenylephrine infusion has developed reflex bradycardia.

39. Vasopressin (Pitressin) may be used for _____ shock.

40. Take a moment to go to the Surviving Sepsis website and check it out! http://www.survivingsepsis.org/Guidelines/Pages/default.aspx

41. List a clinical situation in which midodrine would be indicated.

42. List six clinical signs and symptoms of extravasation.

   a. _____
   b. _____
   c. _____
   d. _____
   e. _____
   f. _____

43. How can the risk of extravasation be minimized?

Inotropic Agents

44. List a clinical indication for dobutamine.

Phosphodiesterase Inhibitors

45. Why would you choose milrinone over inamrinone to manage your patient's hemodynamic status?

Cardiac Glycosides

46. Digoxin, the only drug in the cardiac glycoside class, is used in the management of chronic _____.

47. List four initial symptoms seen in digoxin toxicity.

   a. _____

   b. _____

   c. _____

   d. _____

ELECTROPHYSIOLOGY OF THE MYOCARDIUM

48. List the five major components of the heart's electrical conduction system.

   a. _____
   b. _____
   c. _____
   d. _____
   e. _____

49. When is catheter ablation indicated? What is involved in the procedure? _____

PHARMACOLOGY OF ANTIARRHYTHMICS

50. Quinidine (Quinaglute) is used to treat atrial _____ and _____.

51. Procainamide is indicated in the treatment of _____ _____.

52. Lidocaine is used to control _____ arrhythmias, such as premature ventricular contraction (PVC), ventricular tachycardia, and ventricular fibrillation.

53. A patient with severe asthma is being treated in the cardiovascular intensive care unit (ICU) for hypertension with Lopressor. What is a potential side effect of this medication? Is there a better choice for your patient?

54. In general, amiodarone is used to treat _____ _____ arrhythmias.

55. Class IV drugs such as verapamil (Isoptin) and diltiazem (Cardizem) are referred to as _____-_____.

MANAGEMENT AND PHARMACOTHERAPY OF ADVANCED CARDIAC LIFE SUPPORT

The following is a list of drugs used for advanced life support. Next to the drug give the indication for that drug.

56. Epinephrine: _____

57. Vasopressin: _____

58. Atropine: _____

59. Magnesium sulfate: _____

Answer the following questions.

60. When would intraosseous needle placement be indicated?

61. List the drugs that can be administered through an endotracheal tube (ETT) if IV access is not available.

   a. _____

   b. _____

   c. _____

   d. _____

   e. _____

NATIONAL BOARD OF RESPIRATORY CARE (NBRC) TESTING QUESTIONS

1. Pressure that drives blood into the tissues, averaged over the entire cardiac cycle, is:
   a. Systolic blood pressure
   b. Systemic vascular pressure
   c. Mean arterial pressure
   d. Diastolic blood pressure

2. A patient has a stroke volume of 70 mL/beat and a heart rate of 80 beats/min. What is the CO?
   a. 4.2 L/min
   b. 5.0 L/min
   c. 5.3 L/min
   d. 5.6 L/min

3. Which of the following pressures best evaluates a patient-specific response to fluid therapy and vasoactive therapy?
   a. CVP
   b. MAP
   c. Pulmonary artery pressure
   d. PCWP

4. The normal CO in an adult is:
   a. 8 to 10 L/min
   b. 5 to 7 L/min
   c. 1 to 3 L/min
   d. 10 to 12 L/min

5. Therapies used in the management of shock include:
   1. Fluids
   2. Inotropes
   3. Vasopressors
   4. Cardiac glycosides
      a. 1 and 2 only
      b. 1, 2, and 3 only
      c. 3 and 4 only
      d. 1, 2, 3, and 4

6. Norepinephrine and epinephrine are:
   a. Catecholamines
   b. Inotropes
   c. Calcium channel blockers
   d. Cardiac glycosides

7. Which of the following medications is best indicated for the management of septic shock?
   a. Dopamine (Inotropin)
   b. Vasopressin (Pitressin)
   c. Norepinephrine (Levophed)
   d. Digoxin (Lanoxin)

8. The only cardiac glycoside that is used in the management of chronic heart failure is:
   a. Dopamine
   b. Digoxin
   c. Dobutamine
   d. Epinephrine

9. Which of the following is *not* considered a major component of the heart's electrical conduction system?
   a. SA node
   b. AV node
   c. Bundle of His
   d. Mitral valve

10. Which of the following drugs is used for the treatment of life-threatening ventricular arrhythmias, such as ventricular tachycardia and torsades de pointes?
    a. Quinidine
    b. Procainamide
    c. Lidocaine
    d. Propranolol

11. Which of the following medications is a β-blocker?
    a. Metoprolol
    b. Vasopressin
    c. Magnesium sulfate
    d. Sodium bicarbonate

12. If IV access is not available in a patient with cardiac arrest, which of the following drugs can be administered through an ETT?
    1. Lidocaine
    2. Epinephrine
    3. Atropine
    4. Naloxone
        a. 1 and 2 only
        b. 2 and 3 only
        c. 1, 2, and 4 only
        d. 1, 2, 3, and 4

13. Which of the following statements is *false* regarding the administration of medications through the ETT of a patient in cardiac arrest?
    a. Medications should be placed in the ETT through a catheter that extends beyond the tip of the ETT.
    b. After medication insertion into the lung, 5 to 10 rapid ventilations with a hand-held resuscitation bag should take place.
    c. Chest compressions should continue as drugs are administered through the ETT.
    d. Medications should be diluted with approximately 10 mL of normal saline when they are administered through the ETT.

14. Which of the following is defined as shock?
    a. A mean arterial pressure of less than 80 mm Hg
    b. Organ hypoperfusion and a decrease in oxygen delivery to tissues
    c. A CVP of less than 5 mm Hg and a $Sp0_2$ of less than 90%
    d. A reduction in heart rate less than 60 beats/min and a reduction in CVP less than 5 mm Hg

15. What is the MAP of a patient with a blood pressure of 110/80?
    a. 60 mm Hg
    b. 85 mm Hg
    c. 90 mm Hg
    d. 100 mm Hg

16. When administering medications down an ETT, how much normal saline should be used to dilute the medication?
    a. 5 mL
    b. 10 mL
    c. 12 mL
    d. 15 mL

17. SCD is defined as an episode of which of the following?
    1. Ventricular fibrillation
    2. Pulseless ventricular tachycardia
    3. Pulseless electrical activity
    4. Asystole
        a. 1 and 2
        b. 2 and 3
        c. 1, 2, and 3
        d. 1, 2, 3, and 4

18. What should be done *first* when a patient is in ventricular fibrillation?
    a. IV access
    b. Insertion of an oral airway
    c. Cardiopulmonary resuscitation (CPR) or defibrillation
    d. Insertion of an ETT

19. Which of the following medications would be indicated to increase blood flow to the myocardium and the central nervous system during CPR?
    a. Epinephrine
    b. Atropine
    c. Sodium bicarbonate
    d. Magnesium sulfate

20. Which drug is most appropriate for patients, because of its chronotropic effects, in asystole and can be administered with epinephrine and vasopressin?
    a. Magnesium sulfate
    b. Sodium bicarbonate
    c. Atropine
    d. Vasopressin

CASE STUDY 1

A 19-year-old woman is brought into the emergency department (ED) by ambulance after an automobile crash. The paramedics tell you she has lost a lot of blood. She is intubated and being ventilated with a hand-held resuscitation bag with 100% oxygen. She has IV access.

1. On the basis of this information, what shock state would you suspect?

2. Based on your answer to question 1, how would you expect the following hemodynamic parameters to be altered for this patient?
    a. Blood pressure: _____
    b. Heart rate: _____
    c. CVP: _____
    d. CO: _____
    e. SVR: _____

The patient begins to have multiple PVCs and the doctor orders lidocaine. Her IV was inadvertently pulled out and currently no one has been able to reestablish access.

3. What could you recommend as a route of administration for the lidocaine?

IV access has been reestablished, and a CVP catheter has been inserted. The patient has been treated with various drugs and blood products, and her current hemodynamic parameters are as follows:
   Heart rate: 87 beats/min
   CVP: 9 mm Hg
   Blood pressure: 110/78 mm Hg

4. How would you interpret her hemodynamic status now?

CASE STUDY 2

An 82-year-old (53-kg) woman is in the ED by ambulance from a nursing home. During monitoring of the patient by electrocardiography (ECG) and while applying oxygen, the respiratory therapist recognizes the patient has gone into ventricular fibrillation. The patient becomes unconscious. Shaking and shouting have produced no response by the patient. The respiratory therapist initiates a CODE.

1. What is the first treatment that should be provided to the patient?

2. After this treatment, asystole appears on the ECG monitor. Which drugs would be indicated at this time?

3. What advanced airway could be provided to this patient other than an ETT?

4. After some time of performing CPR, the patient dies. In her chart, the cause of death is SCD. Besides ventricular fibrillation, what other dysrhythmias cause SCD?

22 Drugs Affecting Circulation: Antihypertensives, Antianginals, Antithrombotics

CHAPTER OUTLINE

Key Terms and Definitions
Hypertension
Hypertension Pharmacotherapy
    Angiotensin-Converting Enzyme Inhibitors
    Angiotensin II Receptor Blockers
    Calcium Channel Blockers
Epidemiology, Etiology, and Pathophysiology of Angina
Pharmacotherapy for Angina
    Nitrates
    Ranolazine
Antithrombotic Agents
    Antiplatelet Agents
    Thrombolytics
National Board of Respiratory Care (NBRC) Testing Questions
Case Studies 1 and 2

CHAPTER OBJECTIVES

After answering the following questions, the reader should be able to:

1. Define terms that pertain to drugs affecting circulation: antihypertensives, antianginals, and antithrombotics
2. Categorize the stages of normal to high blood pressure
3. Define a hypertensive crisis and differentiate between hypertensive emergency and urgency
4. Design an algorithm for the pharmacotherapy of hypertension
5. Compare and contrast the clinical pharmacology among the agents used for hypertensive pharmacotherapy
6. Describe the chronotherapeutic effect of blood pressure, and design a pharmacotherapy regimen based on this principle.
7. Describe the mechanism of action of the angiotensin-converting enzyme inhibitors, calcium channel blockers, and β blockers
8. Compare and contrast the clinical pharmacology of spironolactone and eplerenone
9. List antihypertensive relevant drug-drug interactions and plausible mechanisms
10. Describe the formation and elimination of an acute coronary thrombus
11. Describe the pathophysiology of angina and the drugs used to treat angina
12. List the agents in each of the following antithrombotic classes: anticoagulants, antiplatelets, and thrombolytics
13. Compare and contrast the clinical pharmacology of aspirin, clopidogrel, ticlopidine, and dipyridamole
14. Describe the role of genetic polymorphism in the antiplatelet activity of clopidogrel and the anticoagulant effect of warfarin
15. List the indications for and contraindication to thrombolytic agents

KEY TERMS AND DEFINITIONS

Match the following definitions with their terms.

1. _____ Damage to the heart and the blood vessels or circulation, including the brain, kidney, and the eye

2. _____ Maximal dose of a drug, beyond which it no longer exerts a therapeutic effect; however, its toxic effect increases

3. _____ The volume of water filtered from the plasma by the kidney through the glomerular capillary walls into Bowman capsules per unit time

4. _____ Neurotransmitter or hormone replacements that may be weaker or inert

5. _____ Human biologic variations of rhythm within a 24-hour cycle

6. _____ Treatment of disease by drug therapy

7. _____ A drug influencing the contractility of a muscle (heart)

8. _____ Influencing the rate of rhythmic movements (the heartbeat)

9. _____ Drug that prevents or breaks up blood clots in conditions such as thrombosis or embolism

10. _____ Measurement of the renal clearance of endogenous creatinine per unit time

11. _____ Defined hemodynamically as the product of systemic vascular resistance and cardiac output (heart rate × stroke volume)

12. _____ Covalently cross-linked degradation fragments of the cross-linked fibrin polymer during plasmin-mediated fibrinolysis

13. _____ Enzyme also known as *angiotensinogenase* that is released by the kidney in response to a lack of renal blood flow and is responsible for converting angiotensinogen into angiotensin I

14. _____ Blood pressures higher than 180/120 mm Hg, with the elevation of blood pressure accompanied by acute, progressive target organ injury

15. _____ Blood pressures higher than 180/120 mm Hg without signs or symptoms of acute target organ complications

16. _____ Small peptides that result after the action of plasmin on fibrinogen and fibrin in the fibrinolytic process

17. _____ Having the ability to activate and block adrenergic receptors; producing a net stimulatory effect on the sympathetic nervous system

a. Antithrombotic
b. Arterial blood pressure
c. Cardiovascular disease (CVD)
d. Chronotropic
e. Circadian rhythm
f. Creatinine clearance
g. D-dimers
h. Dose-ceiling effect
i. Substitute neurotransmitters
j. Fibrinogen degradation products (FDPs)
k. Glomerular filtration rate (GFR)
l. Hypertensive emergency
m. Hypertensive urgency
n. Inotrope
o. Intrinsic sympathomimetic activity (ISA)
p. Pharmacotherapy
q. Renin

HYPERTENSION

18. List eight pathologies that may result from uncontrolled hypertension.

    a. _____

    b. _____

    c. _____

    d. _____

    e. _____

    f. _____

    g. _____

    h. _____

19. Clay is a 24-year-old male with a history of insulin-dependent diabetes. His blood pressure over the past 6 months has gone from 138/82 mm Hg to 146/88 mm Hg. (a) Should he be treated pharmacologically for his blood pressure? (b) If so, what medication would you suggest?

    a. _____

    b. _____

20. How are blood pressure medications and doses adjusted?

21. Arterial blood pressure is a product of _____ and _____.

HYPERTENSION PHARMACOTHERAPY

Angiotensin-Converting Enzyme Inhibitors

22. How do angiotensin-converting enzyme (ACE) inhibitors work to lower blood pressure?

23. List two common side effects of ACE inhibitors.

    a. _____

    b. _____

Angiotensin II Receptor Blockers

24. How do angiotensin II receptor blockers (ARBs) work to lower blood pressure?

Calcium Channel Blockers

25. List a pathology that may require your patient to be prescribed a calcium channel blocker.

26. Describe the chronotropic effect exhibited by verapamil.

27. Fill in the table with the correct trade names of the generic calcium channel blockers available.

Generic Name	Trade Name
Verapamil	
Diltiazem	
Amlodipine	
Plendil	
Nifedipine	

28. List six symptoms of β-blocker–induced pulmonary dysfunction.

    a. _____
    b. _____
    c. _____
    d. _____
    e. _____
    f. _____

29. Of the five classes of diuretics, which are most commonly used to manage hypertension?

    a. _____
    b. _____

30. List seven common side effects seen with thiazide and thiazide-like diuretics.

    a. _____
    b. _____
    c. _____
    d. _____
    e. _____
    f. _____
    g. _____

31. Your patient is a 31-year-old female with a history of hepatic cirrhosis. What medication would you suggest for treatment?

32. Glenda is a 62-year-old patient who has been taking eplerenone for many years as part of her heart failure and hypertension treatment regimen after her myocardial infarction (MI). She has recently been diagnosed with hyperkalemia and renal insufficiency. Should she be able to maintain her current regimen, or will the physician change her eplerenone to a different medication? Why or why not?

33. How do α_1 adrenergic receptor antagonists lower blood pressure?

EPIDEMIOLOGY, ETIOLOGY, AND PATHOPHYSIOLOGY OF ANGINA

34. List three symptoms exhibited by a patient experiencing angina.

    a. _____

    b. _____

    c. _____

PHARMACOTHERAPY FOR ANGINA

Nitrates

35. How is angina pain relieved with nitrates such as nitroglycerin?

36. If a patient is at home experiencing angina pain, how should he or she take the nitroglycerin?

37. How often should nitroglycerin be administered for relief of angina pain?

Ranolazine

38. What is the indication for ranolazine?

ANTITHROMBOTIC AGENTS

39. List three indications for heparin therapy.

    a. _____

    b. _____

    c. _____

40. Which has a longer time of onset, heparin or warfarin?

Antiplatelet Agents

41. What is a concern when aspirin is given at high doses to patients with asthma and chronic obstructive pulmonary disease (COPD)?

42. List an indication of the use of Plavix.

Thrombolytics

43. List three indications for thrombolytic agents.

    a. _____

    b. _____

    c. _____

44. List two drawbacks seen with the use of warfarin.

    a. _____

    b. _____

45. Fill in the chart relating to new oral anticoagulants.

	Apixaban (Eliquis®)	Rivaroxaban (Xarelto®)	Dabigatran (Pradaxa®)
U.S. Food and Drug Administration (FDA) indication(s)			
Dosing			
Stroke prevention in non-valvular atrial fibrillation			
Deep venous thrombosis (DVT)/pulmonary embolism (PE) treatment			
DVT/PE prophylaxis			
Cautions			
Contraindications			

46. List 10 absolute contraindications for thrombolytic treatment in acute stroke.

    a. _____

    b. _____

    c. _____

    d. _____

    e. _____

    f. _____

    g. _____

    h. _____

    i. _____

    j. _____

NATIONAL BOARD OF RESPIRATORY CARE (NBRC) TESTING QUESTIONS

1. Which of the following is optimal blood pressure for adults 18 years of age or older?
   a. <120/<80 mm Hg
   b. >135/>85 mm Hg
   c. >140/>90 mm Hg
   d. <150/>70 mm Hg

2. Which of the statements is *true* regarding hypertension in adults?
   a. Hypertension is most commonly caused by smoking.
   b. The etiology of hypertension is unknown.
   c. Hypertension occurs less in the United States than other countries.
   d. Hypertension occurs more in nondiabetic patients.

3. Which of the following is the brand name for dabigatran?
   a. Coumadin
   b. Eliquis
   c. Xarelto
   d. Pradaxa

4. Which of the following are hemodynamic effects of ACE inhibitors?
   1. A reduction in peripheral arterial resistance
   2. An increase in cardiac output
   3. An increase in heart rate
   4. An increase in renal blood flow and unchanged GFR
      a. 1 and 2
      b. 3 and 4
      c. 1, 2, and 4
      d. 1, 2, 3, and 4

5. What is the most common adverse effect associated with thrombolytic agents?
   a. Bleeding
   b. Clot formation
   c. Stroke
   d. MI

6. Most MIs, strokes, dysrhythmias, and venous thromboembolic events occur in the _____ _____, in concert with the circadian blood pressure peaks.
   a. Morning hours
   b. Afternoon hours
   c. Evening hours
   d. Relaxation hours

7. Which of the following pulmonary symptoms may occur with the administration of β blockers?
   1. Bronchospasm
   2. Wheezing
   3. Dyspnea
   4. Cough
      a. 1 and 2 only
      b. 2 and 3 only
      c. 2, 3, and 4 only
      d. 1, 2, 3, and 4

8. Of the five classes of diuretics, which are most commonly used to manage hypertension?
   1. Thiazides
   2. Potassium-sparing agents
   3. Adrenergic agents
   4. Antiadrenergic agents
      a. 1 and 2 only
      b. 2 and 3 only
      c. 3 and 4 only
      d. 1 and 4 only

9. How do α_1 antagonists lower blood pressure?
   a. By affecting both cardiac output and glomerular filtration rate
   b. By increasing peripheral vascular resistance
   c. By blocking postsynaptic receptors
   d. By increasing the preload and afterload of the heart

10. Which of the following symptoms are exhibited by a patient experiencing angina?
    1. Chest tightness
    2. Pressure
    3. Burning sensation (indigestion)
    4. Pain radiating to left shoulder and jaw
       a. 1 and 2 only
       b. 2 and 3 only
       c. 1, 3, and 4 only
       d. 1, 2, 3, and 4

11. How is anginal pain relieved with nitrates such as nitroglycerin?
    a. Reduction in cardiac output
    b. Vasodilation of coronary arteries
    c. Peripheral vascular vasodilation
    d. Reduction in platelet adherence to peripheral vasculature

12. A patient with anginal pain was administered a nitroglycerin tablet 5 minutes ago. The patient has had no relief from the pain. What would you recommend?
    a. Seek emergency care.
    b. Wait 30 minutes before taking another nitroglycerin tablet.
    c. Take another nitroglycerin tablet immediately.
    d. Take two nitroglycerin tablets immediately.

13. Which of the following is an indication for heparin therapy?
    1. Prevention of venous thromboembolism
    2. Prevention of coronary artery vasoconstriction
    3. Prevention of platelet adhesion
    4. Prevention of pulmonary vascular vasoconstriction
       a. 1 only
       b. 4 only
       c. 2 and 3 only
       d. 2, 3, and 4 only

14. A patient has been prescribed warfarin. Indications for warfarin include:
    1. Venous thrombosis
    2. PE
    3. Congestive heart failure
    4. Mitral valve stenosis
       a. 1 and 2
       b. 3 and 4
       c. 1, 3, and 4
       d. 2, 3, and 4

15. What is a concern when aspirin is given at high doses to patients with asthma?
    a. It can induce severe bleeding from the gastrointestinal tract.
    b. It can exacerbate asthma symptoms.
    c. Minor bleeding may occur within the pulmonary tract.
    d. It can increase the changes of stroke.

16. Which of the following is a marker or symptom of myocardial ischemia?
    a. Angina
    b. Dizziness
    c. Tingling in the fingers
    d. Double vision

17. Sublingual nitroglycerin tablets lose potency after:
    a. 1 month
    b. 2 months
    c. 4 months
    d. 6 months

18. Which of the following laboratory tests is used to monitor the effects of heparin?
    a. Differential white blood cell count
    b. Activated partial thromboplastin time (aPTT)
    c. Bilirubin urea nitrogen (BUN)
    d. Extended bleed time (EBT)

19. Which of the following are antiplatelet agents?
    1. Enoxaparin (Lovenox)
    2. Warfarin sodium (Coumadin)
    3. Aspirin
    4. Clopidogrel (Plavix)
       a. 1 and 2
       b. 3 and 4
       c. 1, 3, and 4
       d. 1, 2, and 4

20. Primary or essential hypertension is the result of:
    a. Systolic blood pressure increasing 20 mm Hg per hour
    b. Diastolic blood pressure higher than 100 mm Hg
    c. High intake of salt
    d. An unknown cause

CASE STUDY 1

Mrs. A. is a 69-year-old woman with a history of hypertension and angina. She was treated in the hospital 4 months ago for angina with nitrates and an ACE inhibitor. She was sent home with nitroglycerin tablets and told to take one low-dose aspirin a day. This was the only episode of angina, and she has not had angina since then. Early one morning, Mrs. A. got out of bed and was washing her face. Suddenly, she began feeling light-headed with some mild chest discomfort. She turned to her husband and said: "I think I'm having another attack."

1. On the basis of her history, what do you think are Mrs. A.'s symptoms?

2. Mr. A. goes to the medicine cabinet to get nitroglycerin pills. He notices that the pills are 4 months old. Can he still use these pills?

3. Mrs. A. puts a nitroglycerin pill under her tongue. How long before she should start feeling relief?

4. It has been 5 minutes since taking the first nitroglycerin pill, and Mrs. A. has felt no relief from her symptoms. What would you recommend?

5. It has now been 15 minutes, and Mr. A. has given his wife three nitroglycerin pills. Mrs. A. has had no relief. What should Mr. A. do now?

CASE STUDY 2

You are a respiratory therapist working in the emergency department (ED) of a small, rural hospital. Because of the flu, the ED is short-staffed today, so you are assisting in other procedures to help out during this time. Currently, four patients are in the ED:

Patient A is Mr. Wood, a 65-year-old black male.
Patient B is Mrs. Gonzales, a 58-year-old white female.
Patient C is Mr. Alexis, a 55-year-old white male.

Patient D is Mrs. Allen, a 59-year-old black female.
You are asked to take the blood pressure on each patient.

1. Which patient would most likely have hypertension?

After completing the blood pressure measurements on each patient, you record the following:
   Mr. Wood: 150/98 mm Hg
   Mrs. Gonzales: 120/90 mm Hg
   Mr. Alexis: 118/80 mm Hg
   Mrs. Allen: 132/86 mm Hg

2. Which patient would be considered to have hypertension?

On reading Mr. Wood's chart, you see a differential diagnosis of CVD.

3. Why would Mr. Wood have CVD?

4. If Mrs. Gonzales has a heart rate of 70 beats/min and stroke volume of 80 mL/beat of the heart, what would be her cardiac output?

After further evaluating Mr. Wood, the doctor has diagnosed him with uncomplicated hypertension.

5. What are first-line agents that can be used for uncomplicated hypertension?

After completing a physical examination on Mr. Alexis, you have found that he is taking warfarin. Mr. Alexis cannot remember how much of this drug he is taking and when the last time was that he took the drug.

6. What laboratory test can be ordered to determine the level of warfarin?

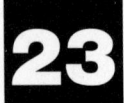 Sleep and Sleep Pharmacology

CHAPTER OUTLINE

Key Terms and Definitions
History of the Treatment of Sleep Disorders
Neurophysiologic Mechanisms
Sleep Disorders: Causes and Treatments
National Board for Respiratory Care (NBRC) Testing Questions
Case Studies 1 and 2

CHAPTER OBJECTIVES

After reading this chapter, the reader should be able to:

1. Define terms that pertain to sleep and sleep pharmacology
2. Describe the definition of sleep, its individual stages, and their electrophysiologic correlates
3. Comprehend the basic neurophysiologic mechanisms that promote brain arousal and wakefulness
4. Comprehend the basic neurophysiologic mechanisms that promote sleep onset and maintenance
5. Describe basic circadian processes and their interaction with the sleep-wake cycle
6. Recognize several sleep disorders that are amenable to pharmacotherapy
7. Describe the rationale for using certain classes of drugs to treat specific sleep-related disorders

KEY TERMS AND DEFINITIONS

Match the following definitions with their terms.

1. _____ Daytime sleepiness that is so great that it leads to inappropriate daytime napping or sleeping

2. _____ A group of sleep disorders manifested by undesirable motor sensory or behavioral phenomena that occur during sleep

3. _____ The approximately 24-hour cycle of biochemical, physiologic, and behavioral processes

4. _____ Compounds that depress central nervous system activity

5. _____ The measurement and recording of electroencephalography (EEG) activity, typically coupled with the measurement and recording of cardiorespiratory activity and eye movements, during sleep

6. _____ The measurement and recording of the gross electrical activity of the brain

7. _____ A class of drugs used to induce sleep

8. _____ Drugs that reduce anxiety and promote muscle relaxation, and also promote sleep

9. _____ Drugs that directly influence circadian mechanisms

a. Parasomnia
b. Electroencephalography
c. Hypnotic
d. Barbiturates
e. Hypersomnia
f. Benzodiazepines
g. Circadian rhythm
h. Chronobiotics
i. Polysomnography

HISTORY OF THE TREATMENT OF SLEEP DISORDERS

Answer or complete the following.

10. Until the mid-1960s, the field of sleep medicine focused primarily on describing and treating insomnia, parasomnias, which include _____ and _____, and hypersomnias, such as _____.

11. The respiratory therapist's role in sleep medicine is still evolving. During the course of a sleep study, what two roles does the respiratory therapist play when working with the physician?

    a. _____

    b. _____

12. The International Classification of Sleep Disorders Revised (ICSD-R) book has identified more than _____ sleep disorders.

13. Perhaps the first compound to be used as a sleep-inducing aid was the juice from the _____ poppy.

14. In the 1800s, Crawford Long, a surgeon in Georgia, employed the recreational drug _____ to induce sleep, amnesia, and pain relief for surgical procedures.

15. Give one reason why nonbenzodiazepine compounds and analogs of these compounds are used instead of benzodiazepine.

16. List three principal characteristics that the ideal hypnotic should possess.

    a. _____

    b. _____

    c. _____

17. List two medications that have been used in an effort to enhance ventilation in patients with high altitude–induced central sleep apnea or obesity-hypoventilation syndrome.

    a. _____

    b. _____

18. Somnambulation or _____ occurs during the first third of the night.

19. Several brain regions are involved in the active process of sleep, especially which two regions?

    a. _____

    b. _____

20. When determining the appropriate pharmaceutical intervention for a sleep disorder, what must be done first?

21. Normal human monophasic sleep has two stages. Name these two stages of sleep.

    a. _____

    b. _____

22. Non–rapid eye movement (NREM) can be categorized into what states of sleep (formerly known as stage 1 to stage 4)?

    a. _____

    b. _____

    c. _____

23. *Match the following concerning sleep stages.*

    1. _____ This stage was formally known as stage 1.
    2. _____ A person is in this sleep stage for 5% to 20% of the total sleep time (TST).
    3. _____ This sleep stage has EEG of relatively low voltage and 20% to 25% TST with lateral eye movements.
    4. _____ TST is 45% to 55%, with no eye movement and low chin muscle activity.
    5. _____ Electromyography (EMG) has high tonic activity, and the patient is in a relaxed wakefulness state.

    a. N1
    b. N2
    c. N3
    d. Awake
    e. Rapid eye movement (REM)

24. A normal sleep cycle begins with sleep stage _____ and proceeds through _____.

25. REM sleep usually first occurs within the first _____ minutes after sleep onset.

26. Adult humans typically sleep about _____ hours per night and spend almost one-third of their life sleeping.

NEUROPHYSIOLOGIC MECHANISMS

Answer or complete the following.

27. List two correlates that arose from observations seen in postmortem examinations of the brains of patients who died from *encephalitis lethargica* after World War I that relate to sleep.

    a. _____

    b. _____

28. Most ascending activation system (AAS) projections that mediate EEG arousal and wakefulness synapse in what brain region?

29. In general, how does sleep begin?

30. List the two components that influence sleep and sleep regulation.

    a. _____

    b. _____

31. Coffee and tea are used ubiquitously to increase alertness, because these beverages contain _____, which is an adenosine receptor antagonist.

32. Circadian rhythms must depend on an internal _____ that is self-sustaining in the absence of external time cues and can be reset by changes in the environment.

33. Localized to the anterior hypothalamus, what brain region acts as the "biological clock" to coordinate the circadian rhythm?

52. _____ are undesirable motor, sensory, or behavioral phenomena that occur primarily during sleep. NREM parasomnia or arousal disorders include confusional arousals, sleep terrors, and sleep walking.

53. What three common factors do primary arousal disorders share?

    a. _____

    b. _____

    c. _____

54. True or False: Sleep terrors are similar to confusional arousals and occur during the first third of the night. Sleep terrors most frequently occur in children aged 5 to 7 years and appear with equal prevalence in boys and girls.

55. _____ or _____ occurs during NREM sleep and is characterized by the presence of automatic behaviors of varying complexity, including walking, eating, mumbling, and, rarely, violence.

56. True or False: The most common pharmaceutical treatment for REM and NREM sleep parasomnias is usually one of the longer-acting benzodiazepines.

57. True or False: A benzodiazepine taken in the evening to reduce the likelihood of experiencing an arousal event may induce residual sleepiness the next day.

NATIONAL BOARD FOR RESPIRATORY CARE (NBRC) TESTING QUESTIONS

1. A patient who is diagnosed with hypersomnia would be treated for:
   a. Sleep walking
   b. Night terror
   c. Narcolepsy
   d. Terror dreams

2. The first compound to induce sleep was the juice from the:
   a. Methadone plant
   b. Opium poppy
   c. Belladonna plant
   d. Eucalyptus plant

3. The modern era of anesthesia was ushered in with the use of:
   a. Ether
   b. Opium
   c. Cocaine
   d. Morphine

4. Although benzodiazepines are considered safe, side effects of these drugs include:
   1. Addiction
   2. Next-day sleepiness
   3. Incontinence
   4. Memory loss
      a. 1 and 2
      b. 2 and 4
      c. 1, 2, and 4
      d. 1, 2, 3, and 4

5. A patient in the doctor's office is being prescribed a hypnotic. If you were the prescribing physician, what would you consider the "ideal" hypnotic to do?
   1. Induce rapid sleep
   2. Maintain sleep over 7 to 8 hours
   3. Have no residual effects on memory
   4. Allow minimal dreams during REM sleep state
      a. 1 and 2
      b. 2 and 4
      c. 1, 2, and 3
      d. 1, 2, and 4

6. Somnambulism occurs during which of the following sleep stages?
   a. N3
   b. N2
   c. N1
   d. Relaxed wakefulness

7. Which of the following neurotransmitters are involved in the production and maintenance of wakefulness?
   1. Histamine
   2. Norepinephrine
   3. Acetylcholine
   4. Anticholinesterase
      a. 1 and 3
      b. 2 and 4
      c. 1, 2, and 3
      d. 1, 2, 3, and 4

8. When people awaken during this sleep state, dream recall is common. This sleep stage is:
   a. N1
   b. N2
   c. N3
   d. REM

9. This sleep stage has a patient exhibiting no eye movement and low chin muscle activity, and the person is in this sleep stage 45% to 55% of the total sleep time. This sleep stage is:
   a. N1
   b. N2
   c. N3
   d. REM

10. REM sleep usually occurs within _____ minutes after sleep onset.
    a. 90
    b. 30
    c. 15
    d. 60

11. Arousal and wakefulness are seen in a person by assessment of which of the following?
    a. Leg twitching
    b. Eye movement laterally and chin movement
    c. EEG
    d. Increased respiratory rate and heart rate

12. You have just pulled an "all nighter" preparing for your pharmacology examination on sleep disorders. You want to stay awake for this examination, so you decide to drink a beverage that is loaded with an adenosine receptor antagonist. Which of the following beverages would you drink?
    1. Coffee
    2. Tea
    3. Cola
    4. Milk (2%)
       a. 4 only
       b. 2 and 4
       c. 1, 2, and 3
       d. 1, 2, 3, and 4

13. In addition to homeostatic need for sleep, sleepiness also depends on another major influence that relies on an internal pacemaker that is self-sustaining and can be reset by influence in the environment. This is referred to as the:
    a. Circadian rhythm
    b. Light/dark rhythm (L/D)
    c. 24-hour light/dark cycle (L/D)
    d. Daytime/nighttime cycle (D/N)

14. Which is a chronobiotic drug that is important for sleep regulation and has been shown to correlate with evening sleepiness?
    a. Levodopa
    b. Melatonin
    c. Dopamine
    d. Adenosine phosphate

15. A patient has come to the doctor's office with complaints of difficulty falling asleep, awakening frequently during the night, and inability to fall back to sleep. During the day, especially while driving, he falls asleep. This patient would have a diagnosis of:
    a. RLS
    b. Narcolepsy
    c. Obstructive sleep apnea
    d. Insomnia

16. A patient who is complaining of excessive daytime sleepiness and cataplexy would be diagnosed with:
    a. RLS
    b. Narcolepsy
    c. PLMD
    d. Insomnia

17. Which of the following is the most diagnosed primary sleep disorder in the United States?
    a. Narcolepsy
    b. RLS
    c. Sleep apnea
    d. Insomnia

18. The onset of narcoleptic symptoms typically occurs between what ages?
    a. 20 and 25 years of age
    b. 15 and 30 years of age
    c. 10 and 20 years of age
    d. 40 and 60 years of age

19. Conservative treatment of narcolepsy involves administration of which of the following medications?
    1. Stimulant for excessive daytime sleepiness
    2. Antidepressant for cataplexy
    3. Hypnotic for insomnia
    4. Hypnotic for fragmented nocturnal sleep
        a. 1 and 3
        b. 2 and 3
        c. 1, 2, and 4
        d. 1, 2, 3, and 4

20. Nonpharmacologic therapies that can be included in the overall treatment of narcolepsy are:
    1. Scheduled naps
    2. Regular sleep and awake schedules
    3. No eating after 6 PM
    4. Eight to 10 glasses of water daily
        a. 1 and 2
        b. 2 and 4
        c. 1, 2, and 3
        d. 1, 2, 3, and 4

21. An undesirable motor, sensory, or behavioral phenomenon that occurs primarily during sleep is called:
    a. REM terror event
    b. NREM hallucination
    c. Parasomnia
    d. REM hallucination

22. A compound that depresses the central nervous system activity and has been used to treat epilepsy is called:
    a. Barbiturate
    b. Long-acting benzodiazepines
    c. Pergolide
    d. Cabergoline

23. NREM sleep parasomnias include which of the following arousals?
    1. Confusional arousals
    2. Sleep terrors
    3. Obstructive sleep apnea
    4. Somnambulation
        a. 1 and 3
        b. 1 and 4
        c. 1, 2, and 4
        d. 2, 3, and 4

24. Which of the following medications would you recommend for a patient diagnosed with RLS who also has had a medical history of hepatic disease?
    a. Pergolide
    b. Levodopa
    c. Ropinirole
    d. Cabergoline

25. Which of the following is the trade name of an immediate-release nonbenzodiazepine that is FDA approved for the treatment of insomnia?
    a. Ambien CR
    b. Rozerem
    c. Lunesta
    d. Restoril

CASE STUDY 1

Mrs. Polaski is in the doctor's office today for a physical examination. Mrs. Polaski is 65 years old, recently widowed, and retired within the past year from public school teaching. Her vital signs are normal, she is slightly overweight, and she has a very low activity level and performs no exercise other than walking her dog in the morning around the neighborhood. During her physical examination, she explains to the physician she feels she has insomnia. The physician asks: "What makes you think you have insomnia?"

1. What symptoms would Mrs. Polaski say she has for her to be diagnosed with insomnia?

2. What else in the patient's history would lead you to believe she has insomnia?

The doctor agrees that she probably has insomnia. Her physician decides to prescribe a 22-mg dose of temazepam (Restoril). She is instructed in the use of the drug and side effects and told if she experiences any of these to call the physician's office.

3. What are the side effects that should be discussed with Mrs. Polaski?

4. After some discussion about the side effects, Mrs. Polaski inquires about how she will know whether the drug is working and what should she expect concerning falling asleep and maintaining sleep throughout the night. What should she be told?

Two weeks after visiting her doctor, Mrs. Polaski calls the physician's office and wants to talk to the doctor about some of her issues with using this drug. She tells the nurse over the phone that since taking the drug prescribed to her, she feels like she is sleepier during the day and because of this has not even walked her dog in the evening. She also states that she seems to be having a greater loss of memory, which she did not have before taking the drug. For example, she puts things down, such as her glasses and cell phone, and cannot remember where she put them. She is also still awakening during the night, although not as much as before taking the drug.

5. What change in medication should be recommended?

6. What are some medications in both immediate-release and modified-release classes that could be prescribed to Mrs. Polaski? (Also include the trade name. You probably have seen these in commercials.)

CASE STUDY 2

Mr. Mart has come to the sleep clinic for an EEG to aid in a diagnosis of a possible sleep disorder. You are the respiratory therapist who will be performing the study. Observing the study is a respiratory therapy student from the local community college who is interested in entering the sleep medicine field. The patient has had the electrodes attached and continuous positive airway pressure (CPAP) mask fitted. The patient is currently in bed, with lights out, and the EEG has begun.

1. The student inquires: "It looks like the patient is not asleep but is relaxed. Is this a stage of sleep, and how do we know he is in this stage?"

2. Another question asked by the respiratory therapy student is: "Are distinct stages seen when a patient sleeps?"

3. The student then asks: "Is there a stage that a person remains in the longest in normal sleep?"

4. The inquisitive student then asks: "How will you know when the patient is in REM sleep?"

5. "OK," the student says, "So what distinguishes REM on the EEG?"